The Scenic Route

Adventures in the Life of a Traveling Nurse

Colleen Lanier

Wasteland Press

www.wastelandpress.net
Shelbyville, KY USA

The Scenic Route:
Adventures in the Life of a Traveling Nurse
by Colleen Lanier

First Printing – October 2013
ISBN: 978-1-60047-912-0
Library of Congress Control Number: 2013951035

Printed in the U.S.A.

0   1   2   3   4   5   6   7   8

To Mom and Dad, who raised me to believe anything was possible if I gave it my best effort. The unshakable foundation you provided allowed me to pursue my dreams wholeheartedly. I love you, admire you, and thank you.

NOTE TO READER

In the interest of preserving the privacy of patients, families, campers, and coworkers, the name of every person in this book has been changed. In some instances, identifying details have been altered in order to protect the confidentiality of patients I have cared for.

The stories and people are real, and the conversations and experiences have been related as truthfully as possible. Any inaccuracies are unintentional.

PROLOGUE

I went on high alert the moment her breathing changed. It was shallower and more rapid than it had been a few hours before, and she seemed restless. I ran through my mental checklist and assessed the situation. I started with the vaporizer, checking to see if it had enough water, and then smoothed her covers, making sure her stuffed animals were tucked in beside her. I took care not to wake her, hoping it would stop before it really got started.

Inching closer, I watched the rise and fall of her chest as I strained for the first sounds of wheezing. I waited patiently, knowing her breathing would tell me everything I needed to know. A few minutes later, I heard a soft wheeze as she exhaled and knew it was time to act.

I left the room quietly and headed down the hall, trying not to wake anyone up. I knocked softly on the door and waited for it to open. When it did, I didn't waste time with a lengthy explanation.

"Betsy."

"Okay." My father nodded and walked me back to my bedroom, his arm resting reassuringly on my shoulder. My little sister was awake now, sitting up, and breathing in the raggedy pattern that told me they would soon be leaving the house. It was a pattern I knew well. I gathered her socks, shoes, and coat, helping my dad get her ready. Once they left, I would not sleep until my mom told me she was okay.

I was eight years old and had already begun my career in nursing.

ALICIA

The Balinese Room was an institution on Galveston Island, built on a pier stretching 600 feet over the waters of the Gulf of Mexico. In its fifty-year history, it had been a nightclub, an infamous gambling hall, and a supper-club. In August 1983, it was a popular restaurant, and my parents and I were enjoying the unobstructed views of the Gulf as we celebrated the beginning of my junior year in college. We were midway through our salads when our tuxedo-clad waiter approached the table, an artificial smile plastered on his face.

"How is everything, folks?"

My father answered. "So far so good."

"Great." He lingered, looking uncomfortable, clasping and unclasping his hands. He turned, took a few steps, and returned to our table.

"Is something wrong....Paul?" I spoke up, hoping I had remembered his name correctly. Paul looked at my father, pointedly ignoring me.

"I don't mean to alarm you, sir, but they just ordered an evacuation of the west end of the island. Would you like your dinner to go?"

I looked at my mom, who looked at my dad. In unison, we looked out the window. There was a hurricane churning in the Gulf, but according to the news that morning, it was several days away. The water was choppy, but the skies were clear.

Mom made the call. "I think we'll be okay to finish dinner."

"Suit yourself. Your entrees should be right out. Don't mind us—we're going to start getting ready for the storm."

"So... nursing school on an island, huh?" My dad laughed.

"At least the trip will be memorable," I said, "and I might get to see Sean sooner than I thought."

I had chosen the University of Texas Medical Branch (UTMB) on Galveston Island, and the fact that my best friend Sean was in

Houston was one of the deciding factors. The other huge plus to UTMB was that nursing school started junior year, so my detour through majors in music, international relations, and history did not put me behind. When school started in a few weeks, we would all be new to the program. My parents had driven me from Chicago with a vanload of my essentials, and the following morning I would be moving into an apartment with two other nursing students. The Balinese Room was our goodbye celebration.

The food was delicious, but it was more than a little distracting to watch the wait-staff take down pictures, remove glassware from the tables, and pack up the bar. Paul didn't offer the dessert menu, and we soon found ourselves back in our hotel watching the news. The west end of the island, which was not protected by the Galveston Seawall, was under a mandatory evacuation order. The rest of the island was encouraged to heed a voluntary evacuation, and people were being urged to leave well ahead of the storm. Our hotel was a block off the Gulf, protected by the Seawall.

At two o'clock in the morning, my mom decided it was time to go, and we went all the way to San Antonio. We played tourist for a day, my mom and I both developed sun poisoning, and we watched the slow approach of the hurricane.

Alicia made landfall about twenty-five miles southwest of Galveston on August 18th, and as soon as the storm cleared Houston, my parents and I were on the road, wanting to get back to the island to see if my apartment had survived the storm.

The drive down Interstate 45 was a lesson in the power of Mother Nature I would never forget. Trees were strewn like matchsticks, and there was a twenty-five-foot fishing boat blocking the right lane of the highway, beached like a whale, no water in sight. Traffic was minimal, and we got back on the island easily, gaping at the sight of downed power lines, piles of debris, and cars displaced by the force of the storm.

We pulled into the parking lot of Casa del Mar and looked up at my apartment, a corner unit on the third floor. A few days earlier, it had a small balcony facing the Gulf, but the balcony was missing, and the sliding glass door led to nothing but sky.

Three stories below my apartment, a burgundy Cadillac was parked along the side of the building. It was an older model, and the passenger side was crushed, buried in the bricks that had peeled off the building. We walked over to take a closer look and stopped short when we saw the bumper sticker: *God is my co-pilot.*

We took pictures of the damaged building, the Cadillac, and a grocery cart sitting in the branches of a tree. The interior of my apartment had fared well, and we were able to unload my possessions before heading back to Houston, where Sean and his parents were expecting me. They had no power, but their home was undamaged. Sean's mom told me they had a freezer full of ice cream, a closet full of board games, and a pool full of tree limbs. I was welcome to stay with them as long as needed.

As we left Galveston, we passed a ten mile line of cars trying to get back on the island. The National Guard had arrived, and access was strictly limited to residents and first responders. Having lived there for less than a day, I had no proof of residency and would not be allowed back on the island for more than a week. By the time I returned, the Cadillac was gone; I never learned who owned it.

I'm Sorry. What?

In the spring of 1985, I started my psychiatric nursing rotation in a locked unit of a small, private hospital. The patients were usually all adults, but as fate would have it, a sixteen-year-old male was admitted because the adolescent wing was full. During shift change, the night nurse reported that he was paranoid, actively hallucinating, and refusing to speak with any of the staff. Smirking, the charge nurse looked at me and said, "He sounds perfect for you, Carlene."

"Colleen."

The staff nurses were not particularly happy about having to deal with nursing students, sometimes gave us assignments they thought would be miserable, and often did not bother to learn our names. This was my third of six days in the unit, and I had yet to see the charge nurse smile.

I found Tim sitting in his room, wedged in the corner as he balanced on the back two legs of a chair. His eyes were closed, and he was humming.

I introduced myself. He did not open his eyes, seemingly unaware of my presence.

"Tim? Can you hear me? I was hoping we could talk for a few minutes."

He tilted his head back against the wall, opening his left eye slightly. He looked me up and down, snorted, and closed his eye.

I stood there, drowning in a very uncomfortable silence. I had learned about the concept of therapeutic silence, but this did not qualify. It was just plain awkward. I had no idea what to do or say and guessed this was why the charge nurse had been smirking a few minutes earlier. I scanned the room, looking for something to talk about. I studied the stack of cassette tapes on his bed: AC/DC, Iron Maiden, Judas Priest, Dio, Metallica, and Ratt. He was clearly a fan of heavy metal music, and that was something I knew quite a lot about. My best friend Sean was the lead singer of a heavy metal band, and I had immersed myself in the genre.

I took a chance. "Dio? I liked *Holy Diver*, but, *come on.* None of these bands can hold a candle to the Scorpions."

Both eyes opened, and I was scanned again. "What do you know about the Scorpions?"

"Try me."

"Lead singer?"

"Klaus Meine."

"Why the Scorpions?"

"The Zoo." I waited, hoping he would engage. "The Zoo" had been a single on their *Animal Magnetism* album, and it was one of Sean's favorites. I had heard it dozens of times and knew the lyrics by heart.

"And?"

"No *and.* 'The Zoo.'"

He seemed satisfied with my answer and leaned forward, dropping his chair onto all four legs. I had his attention and felt a fleeting connection. My triumph was short lived, however, for his expression quickly darkened.

"What?" I found myself holding my breath, hoping he would keep talking.

"Do you now or have you ever worked for the Russians?"

"No. I am Swedish and Norwegian. We stay neutral." I kept a straight face, matching his level of seriousness.

"Big Mac or Whopper?"

"Neither. Quarter pounder with cheese. You?"

"Whopper. Adidas or Nike?"

"Nike. I have wide feet, and they fit better." I saw him glance at my shoes.

Our conversation was succinct, and I let him take the lead. I was trying to establish rapport, the first step in therapeutic communication. That's what my textbook said.

"Are you wearing any listening devices?"

"Just my ears."

"Do you know why I am here?"

"Do you?"

He laughed. "Good one. Wanna listen to some music?"

"Sure."

He closed his eyes, leaned back in his chair, and started moving his head back and forth. The room was silent. I was at a total loss and briefly considered moving my head around to the tune in Tim's head.

I heard a soft whistle and realized we had an audience. The charge nurse was standing in the hallway, and she crooked her index finger, motioning for me to join her. I glanced at Tim, saw he was lost in the music, and left his room.

"Not bad, *Colleen*." She emphasized my name. "Not bad at all. You have to figure out when to push, when to stop, and when to get the hell out. It takes time, but you'll learn. That was a good start."

The next day, I was given the goal of getting him out of his room for at least fifteen minutes. As soon as I entered his room, Tim started asking questions. "Dallas or Dynasty?"

"Dynasty."

"Name two songs off the *Holy Diver* album."

"'Holy Diver' and 'Stand up & Shout.'"

"Best fast food within five blocks of this dump?"

"Schlotzskys. Hands down."

"Still like the Scorpions?"

"Yes. Hasn't changed since the last time we talked."

"Is that your real hair color?"

"Absolutely not. Is that *your* real hair color?" The purple streaks gave it away, but I played along, still working on rapport.

"Absolutely. My mother is an eggplant. Pool or ocean?"

"Ocean. You?"

"Ocean. If people pee in it, it's more diluted."

"Good point. I could use a cup of coffee. Would you join me in the lounge?"

"For fourteen minutes." He grinned, apparently aware of my task. We spent fourteen minutes in the lounge before he stood up and returned to his room, ending our conversation for the day.

On my way out of the unit, I stopped at Tim's door and told him I would see him the following Tuesday. It was the Thursday before Easter, and I had a much anticipated four-day weekend coming.

"Whatever. I'm not going anywhere." He was wedged in the corner, swaying in his chair. He had headphones on, and I could hear Dio singing "Holy Diver." I smiled, waved, and left the unit feeling as if I had, in some small way, connected with him.

I returned to the unit the following Tuesday, well-rested and eager to see if I could get Tim talking. I was curious about the voices he heard and wanted to know what they said to him. I had watched him interact with voices only he could hear and found the concept fascinating. The night shift nurse said he had slept very little and was struggling to adjust to his new medication. He had started on a stronger anti-psychotic Friday afternoon, so this was his fourth day. The day shift nurse, one I had not worked with before, said it could take several weeks to determine if the drug was "a good fit." She warned me to be cautious and to pay attention to his mood.

Tim was not in his room. The room was much tidier, the chair was no longer in the corner, and I did not see his tapes or headphones. It took me a few minutes to find him. He was sitting on a couch along the back wall of the lounge, and it was immediately apparent that things had changed. His posture was rigid, his expression flat, and his hair was stuffed into a knit cap he had pulled right down to his eyebrows. I cautiously approached.

"Hi Tim. It's nice to see you again."

No response. He did not look at me. He was staring at his hands, firmly planted on his knees. He was absolutely still.

I tried again. "How was your weekend, Tim?"

"Tim's not here anymore. I'm Bob."

"I'm sorry. What?"

He repeated himself. "Tim's not here. I'm Bob."

What? I am pretty sure my mouth dropped open. I blinked a few times, failed to come up with an appropriate response, and finally choked out something like, "Could you excuse me? I'll be right back."

I headed directly to the nursing station. I must have had quite an expression on my face because the two nurses stopped talking and looked at me.

"He said, 'Tim's not here. I'm Bob.' I said, 'Hi Tim,' and he said, 'Tim's not here anymore. I'm Bob.'"

They looked at each other, raised their eyebrows, and turned back to me. "And?"

"What am I supposed to do? How do I handle that? What do I say to him?"

"Who says you *can* handle it? If he is Bob now, you have to engage him as Bob. You work with what you are given." They were amused by my confusion, shaking their heads and exchanging a quick roll of the eyes.

"Just talk to him like we've never met? Start over with Bob?" I wasn't clear on how that would work.

"Work with what he gives you. Who's to say Bob isn't the real person? Did you consider that? How do you know who he really is?"

I considered their questions. "I don't know who TimBob is. I don't know if he knows who he is."

My answer got an approving nod from them, and the charge nurse actually chuckled. "TimBob. That's a good one. Look, our job is to help them no matter who they are at any given moment. The name doesn't matter. The person does. It is rarely cut and dried."

"Okay. I'll see what I can do." I returned to the lounge and settled into a chair across from TimBob. "Do you like music, Bob?"

"Not really." He kept his eyes on his hands.

"I like music. A friend of mine sings in a heavy metal band, so I have gotten to know a lot of those bands..." I trailed off, hoping he would jump in.

Nothing. He didn't respond to questions about food, animals, the weather, TV shows, or sports. I got nothing at all, and silence seemed to be our most successful interaction. I shared silence with him until lunchtime, charted my failures in great detail, and was relieved when the day was over.

I had dinner with several of my classmates. Each of us was working on a different psych unit, and everyone had a story to tell. They laughed when I told them about the whole TimBob conversation and particularly liked my less-than-therapeutic reply. "I'm sorry. What?" became a catch phrase that would follow me until graduation.

On Thursday, I returned for my sixth and final day in the locked unit. I had been thinking about new ways to approach TimBob and was feeling up to the challenge. I passed his room on the way to the nursing station. It was empty. A bed had opened in the adolescent wing, and he had been transferred the evening before. I would not see him again. TimBob was gone, and my questions would never be answered.

I was given a new assignment, a woman named Shirley, who was in her early 60's. She had been there many times before, and the nurses knew her well. The charge nurse said, "I think Shirley will like you, Colleen. Just move slowly until she gets used to you, and don't go into her room until you are sure she knows you are there. She doesn't like surprises."

Just move slowly? What? Why? "Okay...anything else?"

"Just see how it goes."

With that less than helpful directive, I headed off to Shirley's room. She was lying in bed with the covers pulled over her head, and I spoke to her from the doorway. "Good morning, Shirley. My name is Colleen, and I am a nursing student. May I come in?"

The covers retracted slightly, and I caught a glimpse of a piercing blue eye behind matted grey hair. Shirley did not speak. She inhaled sharply and let out a piercing scream, her eye disappearing as she pulled the blanket back over her head. I took that as my cue to leave, and as I turned, her scream morphed into a single word: "Diablo!"

The charge nurse was heading down the hall towards Shirley's room as I was beating my rather hasty retreat. Shirley's scream dwindled, and the word became a chant—"Diablo, Diablo, Diablo."

I held my hands up in surrender. "I spoke to her from the doorway, and that was all it took. One look at me, and she started screaming."

The charge nurse patted my shoulder. "Don't worry about it. It will take a while for her meds to kick in, and she probably would have screamed at anyone who approached her."

"Is there anything I should have done differently?"

"No. What works today may not work tomorrow. You just keep trying to find the person behind the screams. Or hallucinations. Or paranoia. It changes every day, and you learn to roll with it."

"Roll with it. *Okay.* I'll look in her chart and see if I can find something to talk about when I try again."

"Sounds good to me. Oh, and Colleen?

"Yeah?"

"We know you aren't the devil. TimBob told us you worked for the Russians." She winked and headed down the hallway. In that instant, I was hooked.

DAVID

The little boy I was looking at couldn't be the right child. I had read the file multiple times because it was hard to believe that the actions described could be true. Surely the child's psychologist had exaggerated, for if the events leading to his arrival were close to being accurate, then my first admission to the child psychiatry unit was a monster.

The six-year-old walking towards me didn't look like a monster, though. He looked more like the type of child that would be picked on at school. He was small for his age, and his oversized glasses swallowed his pale, freckled face. He was clutching his caseworker's hand as they walked down the long hall to the nursing station, and I met them halfway, hoping I was ready.

I had graduated from nursing school two months earlier. It had taken three interviews and a lot of talking on my part to convince the head nurse of an inpatient child psych unit in Galveston that I was up to the challenge and ready to commit to the field. While it was common for new grads to spend a year in general medical-surgical nursing, I had no intention of following that path. Nothing had captured my attention like my time with TimBob, and I knew where I wanted to be. When I graduated, I had a job waiting for me as a staff nurse in child psychiatry. I got exactly what I wanted, and now I was responsible for admitting and assessing this child.

I knelt down to match his eye level and extended my right hand. "Welcome to 3 West, David. My name is Colleen, and I'm one of the nurses. You can call me Nurse Colleen."

He stared at me without blinking, his hands now glued to his sides. His caseworker took a step back, and as I glanced up at her, I thought I saw relief cross her features. It seemed she was more than ready to relinquish responsibility of her young charge. As soon as he spoke, I understood why.

"Are you ready to die?" He still wasn't blinking.

"Not today." I waited.

"Do you know about me—what I am ca-pa-ble of?" He emphasized each syllable, clearly looking for a reaction. I wasn't going to give him one because I knew that the first few minutes would set a tone for his stay.

"I know that you are here so we can help you figure things out and so that you will be safe. I am going to show you to your room, and then we will take a tour of the unit. I think you will like the playground, and by the time we are done looking around, it will be lunch time. There are eight other boys and girls here, and y--"

"I killed them," he interrupted, tilting his head to the right and gazing through lenses that made his eyes look huge. "They made me mad, and I killed them."

"I know." I held his gaze.

"I might kill you." His voice was even, quiet, almost monotone.

"No, David, you won't. Do you want to see your room, or do you want to keep trying to shock me? Your choice."

He laughed and took off down the hall. The unit was one long corridor with rooms on both sides. On one end was the nursing station, positioned next to the door leading out to the playground. The other end of the hallway held the main entrance, which exited into the hospital, a self-contained psych facility. The caseworker hadn't wasted any time in leaving and was closing the main door as David ran towards it.

He was intercepted by Jeff, one of the male staff, who picked him up effortlessly and carried him to his room. I was waiting, and together we unpacked David's belongings, letting him choose the cubby for each item. New admits were put in a single room if at all possible. It could be bumpy the first few days, and we needed that time to evaluate if he could safely share a room or if he could safely have furniture. We started with the bare necessities: a bed attached to the wall, built in cubbies with no removable parts, and a bulletin board. No pushpins, of course, but we encouraged each child to decorate their board with photographs, artwork, or whatever craft could be secured with tape.

David had two photographs in his bag. The first was of his aunt, who had raised him since he was about a year old. His mother had abandoned him, unable to give up the many substances she abused while pregnant. The second picture sent a cold chill down my spine. It was David, smiling at the camera, surrounded by little dogs. I knew all about those dogs. They belonged to his aunt. Well, they used to.

David's aunt had recently been hospitalized, and family members had moved into her home to take care of him. On the fourth day of this arrangement, David carried the dogs to the second floor of the home, and, one by one, he threw them down the stairs. He climbed down the steps, picked them up, and repeated the process. He did this over and over until they were dead and then placed them in his aunt's bed. He was found sleeping in that bed, surrounded by the dogs he had methodically destroyed.

I felt his gaze and looked at him. He looked at me, pointedly looked at the photograph, looked back at me, and smiled. It was a smile devoid of warmth or joy. It was a cold-blooded smile of a child who knew exactly what he had done. Turning his gaze to Jeff, he said, "I'm hungry. Is it almost time to eat? Will you show me where the dining room is? Do you think the other kids will like me? When do we get to go to the playground? I need to take a whiz." He grabbed the front of his pants and hunched forward.

Jeff quickly stepped in. "Nurse Colleen, would you like me to finish the tour? Starting with the men's room?"

"Sounds good. Thanks."

"No problem. Come on, little man. I'll show you where the bathroom is."

David followed him out of the room, turning back to look at me from the hall. "Nurse Colleen, I love you. Will you sit by me at lunch? Please?" He smiled again, and this time it was the smile you would expect from a six-year-old child. Playful, happy, *normal*. It was difficult for me to reconcile the two completely different smiles with the same little boy. I wondered which one was closer to the real David and if he was salvageable or a lost cause at six.

As I reached the nursing station, the charge nurse was hanging up the phone. "Nurse Colleen, can you please take a walk up to the classroom? It seems Rebecca is having a hard time staying on task. Maybe you can help her focus and get back on track."

Those carefully chosen words told me that one of our girls was being aggressive and the teacher needed us to step in and remove her. "On track" was code for "Get up there fast, and get her out. The teacher needs help."

I heard laughter as I passed the community room on my way to pick up Rebecca. It was David, sitting on the couch watching a cartoon with Jeff. He looked happy, at ease, like an ordinary boy. He saw me looking in from the hallway and called out to me.

"Hey, Nurse Colleen, can we have pets here?" He smiled, and for the second time that morning, a chill went down my spine.

ELEVATOR MUSIC

The morning started with a group discussion on assignments for the day. The unit was full, and we had a particularly active group of children. After hearing from the night nurse about multiple disruptions affecting everyone's sleep, Alice, the charge nurse, shook her head and said, "Drink up, everyone. It's gonna be a bumpy day."

I grabbed the coffee pot and handled refills. We drank a lot of coffee on the unit, and the undisputed favorite was Chock full o'Nuts. Dillon, the unit secretary and heart of the unit, was in charge of the coffee fund we all contributed to. She had taken it upon herself to run blind taste tests over the course of several months, and nothing ever beat Chock full o'Nuts. Dillon chose to go by her last name, which always struck me as odd given her habit of addressing the children as "Master" and "Miss." She was just Dillon.

"Colleen," Alice said, giving me first choice, "puppy killer, voodoo, or just plain psycho?" Some of our kids required one-to-one attention, and we rotated coverage in order to avoid burnout and to allow for multiple opinions on each child's triggers and behaviors. It was important to know what was happening with each one of our kids because any one of them could require multiple staff members during a meltdown.

"Psycho, please." Easy choice. Jake was a fascinating kid, and psycho was a fair description. He was the youngest child I had seen with true psychosis, and he kept me on my toes. I liked the challenge and was fond of him. Wary, but fond.

"You got it. He was up most of the night, so maybe he'll be tired enough to have a quiet day."

"I'm sure he'll be a delight. Was he hallucinating, Alice, or just bouncing off the walls?"

"Hallucinations—arms and heads piling up in the corner. The usual. I guess I'll take Mary. I've got a voodoo vibe going on. Jeff, that leaves you with David."

Jeff drained his cup and stood up, filling the doorway with his 6'3" frame. "I like that little guy. There's hope for him. Not enough to let him have pets, of course, but I think he can be salvaged."

"Ok, kids. Let's get our little angels ready for breakfast. Watch for silverware—Billy tried to make it out of the dining room with a fork down his pants last night."

Jeff shook his head. "I need to have a talk with that boy. A spoon maybe, but a fork down your pants? That just isn't a good idea."

I stood up, making a final contribution. "As a general rule, I try to keep utensils out of my pants."

Dillon nodded, pretending to write it down. "Note to self: keep utensils out of your pants."

"Who has what down their pants? Is this anything I need to know about?" The Nurse Manager arrived at the very end of our conversation, his accent unmistakable. Isaac was from the Caribbean and had a wonderful, musical lilt to his voice. He frequently entered the room right as conversations ended and often had a puzzled look on his face, perpetually wondering what his staff was up to based on the few words he heard.

Anyone who did not work in a psych ward might have found our conversation unprofessional and, probably, insensitive. It was a coping mechanism of sorts, I suppose. Our children had horrendous histories and hard-to-comprehend behaviors, and in order to deal with their issues, a dark sense of humor was essential. The day shift was a well-organized, deeply twisted group of individuals who loved these children.

Isaac smiled as I passed him, saying, "Good morning, Colleen. Don't you look...you look...well, you are so very bright today. So blue. In a good way, I mean."

I was very blue that morning. It was 1986, and neon colors ruled. I was wearing an electric blue oversized shirt, a knee-length black skirt, and bright blue nylons. Looking back, it was a prime example of everything wrong about the fashions in the mid to late 1980s. That morning, however, I was feeling stylish and "bright."

"Thanks, Isaac. Dillon will fill you in. We have decided to keep utensils out of everyone's pants today."

"Dillon?" I heard Isaac start to question her as I headed for the community room to help with breakfast.

Meals were served on the unit, and staff ate with the children. No time was wasted in getting settled at the table because transitions created opportunities for acting out behaviors. My many years of waitressing came in handy, and the kids seemed to think it was cool I could balance so many plates at once. Mealtimes were a group effort, and we worked hard to make them run smoothly. Each time we sat down to eat, we attempted to control the pace and model appropriate manners including, in some cases, the use of napkins, spoons, and forks.

All of the kids made it to the classroom that morning, and I had almost an hour to chart and work on the weekend activity schedule before getting the call that I was needed upstairs. The classrooms were a floor above our ground floor unit, accessible by elevator or stairs. It could be tricky to get an out-of-control child back to the unit, and the choice between stairs or the elevator was carefully considered.

I paused outside the classroom door, out of the children's line of sight but visible to the teacher. She caught my eye and made a quick gesture with her left hand, a swooping motion upwards, telling me that he was escalating. Jake, the child I had chosen, was known for violent outbursts when his escalations were not diffused. I entered the room quickly and put myself between Jake and the nearest child. I picked up a crayon and put it back in the box, straightening the table as a cue to him that we were wrapping up that activity. His paper was covered in red crayon, and, on closer inspection, I saw it was a drawing of severed heads floating in a bathtub.

Jake was schizophrenic and came to us after suffering a psychotic break during which he had attacked his family. He was seven when admitted to the unit and had been hurting his mother since he was four. She broke down during his intake, telling us she feared he would eventually kill someone. He didn't care that he hurt people and had no remorse. It wasn't long before he hurt me, and I saw exactly what his mother was talking about.

Jake hallucinated, and in spite of several anti-psychotic medication trials, his hallucinations persisted. They happened mostly during the night, and when he chose to tell us what he was seeing, it was almost always severed body parts. He would relay this information in a dispassionate voice and then ask to be tucked in. The first time I tucked him in, he looked up at me, said "Thank you, Nurse Colleen," and punched me square in the eye. His expression never changed. No warning, no remorse. His mother, who I never saw after his admission, was right about her son. The angelic looking seven-year-old with tousled brown hair and innocent eyes would strike without hesitation.

"Jake, time to head back to the unit. You have a visit with Dr. Sam in a few minutes, so we'll go down together."

Jake got up, wordlessly, and walked out into the hallway. There was a stillness around him that was not comforting. It was more of a calm-before-the-storm type of feeling. I looked at the teacher and then the phone. She nodded, picked it up, and let the unit know we were on the way down. While Jake did not seem to be responding to any of the medications, we had gotten better at reading him and sensing when he was going to snap. More often than not, we were able to diffuse the escalation by removing him from the situation.

I did not want to risk the staircase, so we headed for the elevator. I let him push the button, and he pressed himself against the doors as if wanting to go right through them. We had to wait for a minute or two for the elevator to arrive, and he started to bounce on the balls of his feet, another indicator of agitation.

When the doors finally opened, he squeezed between them and turned towards me, eyes dark and cold. The quietness was gone, and he launched at me as I entered the elevator, his arms outstretched toward my face.

I was ready for him, grabbing both wrists, stretching his arms above his head, and turning him around so he was facing away from me. I crossed his arms in front of him, pulled him up against me and slid down the elevator wall, bringing us both into a sitting position on the floor. A classic basket hold, the safest way to restrain a child, and the most commonly used hold on our unit. It was a move I had used many times before. He was contained, neither of us was hurt, and we could ride down to the first floor and try to salvage his day.

It had happened very quickly, and while I was pleased at how nicely we had settled onto the floor, I realized that we had a small problem. I hadn't had time to hit the button for the 1st floor, and now I couldn't reach it. We weren't going anywhere, not until someone called for the elevator or the unit figured out we were taking too long. For the time being, I was going to stay exactly where I was, sitting on an elevator floor, my electric blue legs splayed out before me with a silent, psychotic child held firmly in my grip.

An unexpected quiet in the middle of my shift, exactly what Jake needed. There was nothing to agitate him, no distractions, and he seemed to be relaxing. I could feel the tension leave his shoulders; he leaned back into me and, to my amazement, started to hum. It wasn't a tune I recognized, but it was a pretty good impression of Muzak. I was smiling behind him, and within a few minutes, the elevator started moving. It went down, stopping one floor below.

The doors slid open, revealing Isaac and Dr. Sam. Isaac got that puzzled look on his face, and Dr. Sam just stared. I thought perhaps one of them might offer some assistance, but neither seemed inclined to move. They just stared down at us, and we remained on the floor. The doors started to close.

"Isaac, hold the door please. Could you ask Jeff to join us for a moment?" I was going to need help getting Jake out of the elevator and wasn't going to take the chance of letting him take a swing at me while I was on the floor. I knew better.

"Let me help you, Colleen." Isaac stepped in the elevator, reaching down and putting his hands on top of mine so I could release Jake's wrists into his custody. It did not go smoothly, however, not too surprising given that Isaac rarely participated in takedowns. He was a good manager but never seemed entirely comfortable interacting with the kids. Jake got both hands free, reaching forward to claw at my legs still splayed out on the floor. I was able to grab his arms and pull him back into a basket hold, but my neon blue nylons paid the price of the failed transfer. As I repositioned him against me, I saw long rips in both legs of my nylons. I had a fleeting moment of silence for my now-defunct hosiery.

Isaac had quickly retreated from the elevator, giving me room to maneuver. Dr. Sam had gone next door to the unit to find help, and I saw him coming back with Jeff. Jake was looking at my legs and laughing. My skin peeked out, glaringly white against the neon blue, and I decided I needed to rethink my wardrobe.

Jake stopped laughing and went still. I felt the tension building in his body, and carefully adjusted my grip. He spoke quietly, almost plaintively. "Isaac?"

"Yes, Jake?" Isaac squatted down to eye level, giving Jake his full attention from the safety of the hallway.

In a perfect imitation of Isaac's Caribbean accent, Jake said, "Blow it out your ass, Mon. We were enjoying the music."

I saw Jeff double over, and I bit my lip as hard as I could, willing myself not to burst out laughing. As Isaac remained squatting, seemingly frozen, the elevator doors slid shut, and Jake and I were once again alone. He started humming, and we both enjoyed the music.

Things They Don't Teach You
in Nursing School

"Nurse Colleen, Nurse Colleen! I need some grease. I need it now!" The excited voice carried down the hall, reaching the nurse's station before the child did.

"Grease? Slow down, Ryan. I don't understand." Ryan had just returned from a four-hour visit with his parents. It was Saturday afternoon, and we were hoping that he would be ready for discharge by the end of the week. He had been smiling when his father dropped him off a few minutes earlier, but he wasn't smiling now.

"I need grease, Nurse Colleen! I had pop-pops for lunch, and I need grease. Hurry! Hurry! I need it now." He was clutching his abdomen, jumping from one foot to the other, panic written across his face.

"What kind of grease are you talking about, Ryan?"

"Grease! You know, the stuff in a tub." One of Ryan's diagnoses was pica, meaning he had compulsive cravings to eat non-food items. He gravitated towards dirt, crayons, and toilet paper, though, so his request for grease didn't make sense to me.

"Why do you need grease?"

"I ate pop-pops, Nurse Colleen! Lots of them, and now I have to go. I need it bad." He was twisting the front of his shirt, continuing to hop from foot to foot.

As so often happened, Dillon saved the day. She hung up the phone, opened a drawer, and held up a tub of Vaseline. She winked at me as she passed, steering Ryan down the hall. "Nurse Colleen is a Yankee, Master Ryan. She doesn't know about pop-pops. Let's find Jeff, and get you to the bathroom."

Pop-pops? I had no idea what either one of them was talking about or why Vaseline was involved. Dillon set me straight when she returned, laughing at my confusion.

"Pop-pops are fried jalapenos, Colleen. The hotter the better. Problem is, they come out as hot as they go in. He wanted to grease his bottom so it wouldn't hurt when he pooped. Smart boy. Jeff will make sure he doesn't eat it. The Vaseline, I mean."

I laughed. "And why do you have a tub of Vaseline in your desk, Dillon?"

"Because I like pop-pops, too. Always prepared, Colleen, always prepared."

JANUARY 28, 1986

The first twenty minutes of my shift were spent sitting on the floor of the Quiet Room with a raging child's incisors clamped onto the fleshy part of my right palm. It wasn't comfortable, and I was almost past the point of being amused by the string of rather colorful profanity coming out around his tightly-clamped teeth. Almost, but not quite. Charlie, recently dubbed Chomping Charlie, was one creative five-year-old.

The Quiet Room was directly across from the nursing station and was, in essence, a padded cell. It was about 6 feet by 8 feet, and every inch was covered with tan vinyl over industrial-strength padding. The door locked from the outside and had a small square window that started five feet up. I found the window challenging because I was exactly five feet tall. I had to stand on my tip-toes to peer in when a child was inside. A child could request time in the room or could be escorted there until able to control themselves enough to be safe.

This morning had been an escorted excursion to the Quiet Room, the result of Charlie's unprovoked attack on his roommate.

The standard procedure for getting out of the room was to sit quietly against the back wall for five minutes. That time started when the staff person left the room. I would not be leaving until my hand was released by his teeth, so the clock was not yet ticking.

"You know what I'm gonna do, Nurse Colleen?"

"I hope you're going to stop biting me so we can get on with our day."

"Wrong. I'm gonna bite you until you bleed so much we both f-ing drown. We're going to drown in your blood. Take that, Bitch Colleen." He was hissing through his teeth, and I could feel his saliva dripping down my hand. I knew I would be free soon and sat tight.

"Sorry to disappoint you, Charlie, but I don't have enough blood to drown in. I have a gallon-and-a-half tops, and that won't even cover the floor. You need a new plan, my friend."

He paused for a moment, bit a little harder, and offered Plan B. "I am going to shove icicles up your ass until you shit popsicles. I'll do it—you watch."

"Charlie, we're in Texas. Where will you get icicles? I don't think you thought this through. Any other ideas this morning, or are you done?"

"You make me so mad! Stop talking! Stop talking! Your voice makes my ears bleed! I hate your stupid Yankee guts. You are a stupid Yankee—I heard all about you being born in stupid Michigan. All the people born in Michigan are stupid Yankees. You are so stupid your parents tried to give you a brain transplant." His voice trailed off as he was forced to swallow the saliva created by his yelling, and I had my window of opportunity. I pushed my hand into his mouth as he swallowed, and the action took him by surprise, causing him to open his mouth. I was free, and he was wrapped up in a basket hold before he had a chance to struggle.

I spoke loudly towards the door. "Okay—we're ready."

Jeff's face appeared in the window, and I nodded as he raised an eyebrow, letting him know I was ready to let him step in with Charlie. He opened the door, and we changed positions as we talked. "Charlie is having a rough morning, Jeff. Seems his roommate looked at him with evil eyes, and Charlie decided to bite him. My hand got in the way, so we came down here to calm down and get our day back on track."

"The evil eye, huh? I hate when that happens. I gotta be straight with you, Charlie. Biting Nurse Colleen wasn't your best choice." Jeff's conversational approach worked well with the kids, making them feel as if he were commiserating with them. "Let's sit here a few minutes and decide how to handle it for next time. Life is full of evil eyes. Hate those evil eyes, but life is full of them."

Charlie was now sitting beside Jeff along the back wall, nodding his head in agreement as Jeff spoke. Jeff had his arm around Charlie's shoulders, loosely gripping his wrists, ready for whatever came next: restraining him or backing off and letting him earn his way out of the Quiet Room. I left, closing the door behind me and headed to the nursing station, rubbing my right hand. A single drop of blood appeared in the outline of Charlie's right front tooth.

"Well played, Colleen. Talk until his ears bleed." Dillon greeted me with a smile, alcohol wipes, and a cup of coffee. "I think that popsicle comment might make it into the book." The book was a spiral notebook the staff had started years before, containing statements made by our kids. We didn't want to forget what they said, and many of the comments were hilarious. I had added more than a few during the past year and agreed that Charlie had earned a few lines that morning.

"Not the best way to start the morning, Dillon. Did someone grab my purse?" I had just entered the unit when Charlie saw the evil eye and did not have time to do anything other than drop my things and wade into the fray. I let Charlie's face get too close to my hands, and he bit me. As I carried him down the hall, I had stepped on my purse, inadvertently causing some of the contents to spill onto the floor.

"Of course. Can't let our chilluns get their little hands on the weapons in your bag. Good stuff in there: pen, nail file, a couple barrettes. Everything's in the file cabinet safe and sound. I helped myself to some Tic Tacs, though. They looked good."

"Thanks, Dillon. Always good to be minty fresh."

She laughed. "I think the kids are wound up because of the launch. They have been talking about it all week, and I know they are excited to watch. My sons are. They'll be watching it from school."

"You're probably right. Things should calm down this afternoon."

I headed down to the community room. Breakfast was in progress, and there was an excited buzz in the room. Miss Temple was the lead teacher and had joined us because class was being held on the unit today. We had a much bigger screen than the one in the classroom. Miss Temple had done a great job in engaging the kids' interest in the launch of the Space Shuttle Challenger. The fact that a teacher was going into space was a big deal, and we had decided to hold a launch party.

After breakfast, we let the kids have sixty minutes on the playground so Miss Temple and Brenda, her aide, could set up the room. We had a good time and let them blow off a lot of steam. With the exception of a few bugs being squashed and Ryan eating some dirt, it was uneventful.

By the time we returned from the playground and washed up, the community room had been transformed into a theater. Miss Temple reviewed the planets, the parts of the shuttle, and what we would see as the shuttle reached orbit. The kids had painted pictures of the shuttle and took turns taping them to the walls. By 10:00 am, the walls were covered, each child was in their "launch chair," and we started the thirty-minute countdown along with CNN.

We joined in on the final countdown, starting with "ten… nine…eight… seven…six." At six seconds, the engines ignited, and red flames appeared. The kids responded.

"Cool!"

"Awesome!"

"Wicked!"

The Space Shuttle Challenger launched at 10:37 am, and we cheered. Miss Temple was peppered with questions.

"Why aren't the flames red anymore?"

"Why is the fire black now?"

"All I see is white smoke. Can the astronauts see through all that smoke?"

"Why is it flying sideways?"

A few of the kids were silent, their eyes glued to the screen. We all watched, cheered, clapped, and tried to answer the overlapping questions.

And then it happened. 10:38 am. The explosion. The screen filled with the sights and sounds of the disaster, the two divergent plumes of white, and then silence.

The broadcasters were silent. The room was silent. We stared at the screen, and after what felt like an eternity, a lone voice from the tower said, "Flight controllers here are looking very carefully at the situation…obviously a major malfunction."

Those three words hung in the air before sinking in. A major malfunction. Jeff, Miss Temple, and I looked at each other, stunned, and then started damage control. Jeff turned off the TV, and we tried to divert their attention back towards the kitchen area, away from the television. We did not succeed, and the children started to react.

"A major malfunction, a major malfunction." It was David, yelling at the top of his lungs, running in circles and mimicking explosions by thrusting his arms and legs out widely, shaking his whole body. "Kaboom! Major malfunction! Boom! Boom! Major malfunction!"

Jake ran to the window, craning his neck to look straight up. "Where is it? Where is it? Where are they?" His agitation was increasing rapidly. He had his body pressed against the floor to ceiling window, his outstretched palms pushing against the glass.

Mary had curled into the fetal position, sucking her thumb and moaning softly. Chomping Charlie was jumping up and down yelling, "Cool! I want to see it again. Let's watch it again. That was so cool. I'll bet they're dead. Are they dead, Nurse Colleen? Can we watch it again?"

Several of the kids seemed oblivious to what had happened, and Dillon herded them into the hallway for a game of indoor bowling. The oversized, foam bowling pins were always a hit, and as calm was not possible, organized activity was a great option. She had three kids in the hall, leaving six for Jeff, Miss Temple, Brenda and me. Isaac was off the unit for a meeting, and it was clear we needed help. Quickly.

I dialed the conference room, my hands shaking. "Interrupt the meeting. The kids just watched the Challenger explode on live TV, and we are in trouble down here. We need all hands on deck NOW. Run, okay?"

"Will any of their heads land here? Where are their heads? I can't see them. Nurse Colleen, can we go outside and look?" Jake had left the window to grab my hand, trying to pull me towards the playground door. His face was contorted, and I knew he was on the edge of losing control.

Miss Temple stepped in, trying to help me slow Jake's spiral until reinforcements arrived. "Jake, the shuttle was in Florida, at Cape Canaveral. Remember when we looked at the map? Can you help me put the chairs back around the tables? I could really use your help."

I decided that divide and conquer was our best hope. "Jeff, can you carry Mary to the girls' room?" Mary, still curled into the fetal position, offered no resistance as Jeff scooped her off the floor.

"Brenda, take Christine's hand, and go with Jeff. Please keep those two in their room. Read, color, sing, silence…whatever works. Just keep the door open and call if you need help." Brenda looked at me, nodded, and took the hand of the sobbing nine-year-old, leading her down the hall.

Miss Temple had Charlie near a table, asking him to draw what he saw. He couldn't stop moving long enough to use paper but had a crayon in hand, drawing in the air with wide, jerking motions.

David had not stopped shouting; his cries of "Major malfunction" interspersed with the sobs and shouts of other children. It was mayhem, but we were maintaining safety, and only Jake seemed headed for a complete meltdown. He was back at the window, looking for falling body parts. I wondered if this came close to his hallucinations.

Isaac, Dr. Sam, and a child therapist arrived, their faces flushed from running. They stood in the doorway of the community room, listening, scanning, and trying to get a sense of what was happening and who needed what. Isaac looked at me, silently giving me the lead to direct traffic.

"Dr. Sam, Jake is concerned that body parts will be landing outside the unit. Could you take him out to the playground? You probably want to bring someone else to help you look." It wouldn't be safe to take Jake out alone but letting him hunt for body parts was our best hope for calming him, and I hoped that two of them could handle him. Jake launched himself down the hall with Dr. Sam and a therapist in his wake.

Miss Temple joined Dillon in the hallway, and Isaac went room to room, checking on all of our kids and helping as needed. Jeff had returned from carrying Mary to her room and took David to the Quiet Room so he could continue to yell and flail in a safe environment. David responded well to the confines of the Quiet Room and often asked to go in when he felt out of control.

Charlie and I were alone in the community room. He was agitated but not escalating, more excited than anything else. I could see Jake and Dr. Sam inspecting the ground and looking up into the sky, pointing towards Florida. Jake was searching very thoroughly, looking under bushes, benches, and swings.

"Nurse Colleen, doesn't Jake know they burned up in the sky? What does he think he will find under that bench?" Charlie had stopped circling the room long enough to stand beside me, watching Jake and Dr. Sam scour the playground. His mood shifted quickly as he focused on Jake.

"He needs to look, Charlie. It's important to him." As we stood at the window, I offered Charlie my right hand, the same hand he had recently bitten, and was pleasantly surprised when he took it, squeezing it and pressing a cheek against my forearm.

He spoke quietly. "I just don't get that kid. He's out there. You know what I mean?"

I did indeed.

"Nurse Colleen?"

"Yes, Charlie?"

"Do you think God opened the door when the shuttle exploded?"

"Do you?" I waited. He looked thoughtful.

"They were close to Heaven. God likes astronauts and teachers. I think he opened the door and let them in."

The wisdom of children never ceased to amaze me. "I'd like to think that's exactly what happened, Charlie. How about we draw that so you can show the other kids?"

"Okay. Some of these little kids probably don't understand." My five-year-old charge grabbed some crayons and started drawing. I could hear David yelling, Christine sobbing, and cheers coming from the bowling tournament. For reasons I did not understand, Jake had started digging a hole. The clock chimed on the quarter hour, and I registered the time.

It was 11: 15 am, and our day was just getting started.

THE AFTERMATH

I had no time to think about what had happened that morning. The kids remained agitated, feeding off each other and making it very difficult for us to find any sense of calm. We did the best we could, giving the kids leeway as they each dealt with the explosion in their own unique way. We had tantrums, obscenity-laden diatribes, lots of tears, and complete withdrawal.

My eight-hour shift felt like days, and I was relieved to see Ellen, the evening nurse, come through the doors. We walked the unit, talking about each child's reaction and "taking the temperature" as she called it. Ellen had been a psych nurse for almost thirty years, and nothing seemed to faze her. Nothing until today, that is. Today she was different, and I could feel a sadness rolling off her.

"You okay, Ellen?"

"I watched it with my grandson this morning. Jeremy, you know, the one that wants to be an astronaut? When I left for work this afternoon, he asked me if my car was going to explode."

"I'm sorry, El. It must have been hard to see that fear on his face."

"It's not just that, Colleen. It got me thinking. What if today was the last day I had? I would leave so many things undone. You know how many years I have been saying 'next year' when it comes to vacations, doing something different, trying something new? I've been working in this building for twenty-one years. It's been 'next year' for decades now. What if it's too late?"

I was silent.

"Do something for me, will you?"

"Of course," I answered without hesitation. "Anything, El."

"Don't stay here for twenty years. Go out, and do everything you possibly can. You know that ad you showed me? Don't just look at it; do it! You would be great."

Our conversation was interrupted by a loud moan coming from the girls' room, the last stop on our tour of the unit. It was Mary, still curled tightly into the fetal position, and moaning at intervals. The sound was unlike any I had heard before—ethereal and eerie.

"I think we're finally going to see one of her spells, Ellen."

"I was beginning to wonder if she really had them," Ellen said. "This should be interesting. We'll talk later, okay? Don't worry about me."

I gave her a quick hug, dropping the subject of missed opportunities and getting back to Mary. "Today may be the day you meet Voodoo Mary, El."

Mary was very small for a nine-year-old. Social services had become involved with her family when her absences from school became excessive. The family had explained that they kept her out of school when she had a "spell" and that these spells were the result of her being "touched with the gift." Her spells reportedly lasted days to weeks, and her extended family would gather, waiting to hear what she said when she "returned" from the other side. The family, whose roots went back several generations in Louisiana, believed in Voodoo and practiced many of its traditions.

These spells apparently took a toll on Mary, and the state had taken temporary custody due to malnutrition, truancy, and failure to thrive. She was brought to us with the expectation that the psychiatric staff could diagnose her and offer a treatment plan. Mary had been with us for a week and a half, and we had seen nothing unusual.

"She'll still be here tomorrow, Colleen. Go home, relax, and hug someone."

I trudged out to my car, glad to be heading home to a quiet apartment. I put my purse on the seat beside me and noticed the magazine open to the ad Ellen had just mentioned: *Travel nurses needed.* It was an ad I had first noticed when I was still in school, and the idea of being paid to travel around the country while working as a nurse seemed almost too good to be true. I had been fascinated by maps for as long as I could remember, and actually living in the places I had looked at was very appealing. I kept the idea in the back of my head, thinking that someday I might give it a try.

Ellen's words had struck a chord with me, and I started planning instead of just thinking.

* * * *

Several months later, we were no closer to diagnosing Mary than we had been the day she arrived. We had seen multiple spells, which involved her becoming non-verbal and exhibiting bizarre behaviors such as gulping from the shower head until she vomited, refusing to eat, drinking from the toilets, and biting her lips until they bled. Her posture changed, and she shuffled her feet, hunching her shoulders forward and holding her hands up against her chest, curling her fingers like claws. It reminded me of a praying mantis.

Mary had been transferred to a pediatric medical floor three times for IV hydration and correction of electrolyte imbalances from water intoxication. The pediatric nurses were not comfortable having her on the floor without backup from psych, so we took turns staying with her in the main hospital. She had been transferred back to our unit a few days earlier, and we hadn't seen a spell since her return.

I was working the overnight shift, and Jeff was the second person, having picked up an extra shift when someone called in sick. Night shift was just two staff, and we found ourselves sitting in the hall outside the nursing station, chatting softly and doing paperwork between bed checks. The kids were checked every fifteen minutes at night, and we took turns making rounds and keeping our coffee cups full of freshly brewed Chock full o'Nuts.

1:29 am. I had just looked at the clock and was standing up to make my rounds when we heard it. A laugh and a thud followed quickly by a second thud. We headed down the hall, trying to place the location of the sounds. It was the girls' room; it was Mary.

"Oh my God...look at her." Jeff spoke quietly, almost a whisper, as we came face to face with a version of Mary we had never seen.

She was sitting cross-legged on her bed, laughing, and hitting her head against the wall. Her eyes were opened wide, showing the whites far more than normal. Her laugh raised the hairs on the back of my neck.

"Mary. You have my attention. Enough." I approached her slowly, giving her the opportunity to stop on her own.

She stopped laughing but didn't speak. She looked at us, smiled, and hit the wall even harder, causing both Jeff and I to intervene. We had done enough holds together to know exactly what the other person would be doing, and in a few well-coordinated seconds, we had her on her back, lying on the floor, a pillow under her head to prevent further head banging.

This was not an ordinary hold, however, and even though we were both holding her, Jeff at her knees and me at her shoulders, the three of us were moving. She was moving us across the room, slowly but surely, and I had no idea what to do. The look on Jeff's face told me he was equally at a loss.

"Mary," I spoke quietly, not wanting to wake any of the other children. "I need you to stop moving and relax. We want to let you go so you can get back to bed. Everyone else is sleeping, and this is not the time for this. Work with me, please."

She was silent, her eyes wide open but vacant. She undulated in a subtle wave-like motion, and the three of us, inch by inch, moved towards the door. There was no way it should have happened. We outweighed her 4:1, and yet she was moving us. Time for Plan B.

"Jeff, let's see if she will hold still if we let go." He nodded, and I released her shoulders, moving into position above her head, ready to step back in if needed.

Jeff spoke quietly. "Mary, it's time to get back to bed. I'm going to let go of your legs, and I want you to show me you can be safe. When I let go, I want you to lie quietly. 3, 2, 1." Counting down was a common practice, and he let go at "one." In a split second, Mary knocked the pillow out of the way. I was ready though and got my hands between her head and the tile before she could hurt herself.

Jeff and I held Mary for a total of forty-three minutes. She managed to turn us in a 360-degree circle, and, in spite of our efforts, we ended up in the hallway outside the girl's bedroom. At 2:15 am she stopped moving and went to sleep on the floor. Jeff and I looked at each other, and I shook my head, at a loss for words.

"Soooo...how do you plan on charting this, Colleen?"

"Honestly, I have no idea."

"Well, good luck with that." He released Mary's legs and moved away.

"I'll stay with her while you make rounds. Grab her blanket, okay?"

He handed me her blanket and I covered her, sitting on the floor until I felt it was safe to move her. Shortly after 3 am, Jeff carried her back into her room. She slept through until morning.

We tried to convey the intensity of our experience to the morning shift, but no one truly grasped what had happened, probably thinking we were exaggerating. Not a surprising response, given that it sounded unbelievable. Jeff was 6'3" and close to 200 pounds. Mary tipped the scales at about sixty. Jeff walked me to my car, and we stood by my trunk for a few minutes, trying to put our thoughts into words.

He spoke first. "How in the hell did that child move with both of us holding her down? There's no way that should have happened."

"I know, but it did, and I don't think anyone believed us. I'm glad I wasn't alone with her, you know? She scared me."

"I hear you. Freaked me out, and that's not easy to do. Every time I think I've seen it all, one of these kids lets me know I'm wrong. Totally wrong. You're going to miss this, Colleen. I know you will. You're going to miss these kids."

"Of course I will. There are lots of child psych units out there, though, and it's time for me to go."

Travel nurses needed. I had answered the call.

* * * *

Interestingly, Mary never showed any out of the ordinary behaviors again. She was discharged back into her parents' care a few weeks later with the diagnoses of electrolyte imbalance, malnutrition, and failure to thrive. We had no answers.

TRAVEL NURSING

When I graduated from nursing school in 1985, a nursing shortage was in full swing, and jobs were plentiful. Each of my classmates had multiple job offers to choose from as hospitals scrambled to fill open positions. In response to this need, the industry of travel nursing was born. The concept was simple. Hospitals needed nurses, and nurses wanted options. An experienced nurse was contracted on a short-term basis to fill temporary, seasonal, or unanticipated staffing shortages.

Travel nurse agencies served as brokers, matching hospital needs with available nurses. As a travel nurse, you had the freedom to choose where you worked, what hours you worked, and how long you wanted to stay. The standard contract was thirteen weeks, but it was easy to extend your stay if you wanted to. The travel nurse agency handled all the details and provided housing, travel expenses, and incentives to book multiple assignments with them.

I looked into multiple agencies before choosing the one I wanted to work with. My agency was in Boston, and my recruiter was named Keri. She was organized, easy to work with, and friendly. When I was ready for an assignment, she would tell me every opening they had in my specialty and give me details on any I was interested in. I would look at the map for a while, decide where I would like to go, and call her back to set up an "interview." The interviews were a formality, and the only topic consistently discussed was what shift I was willing to work.

I was approved for work in pediatric and adult psychiatry units, pediatric rehab, and general pediatrics. I'd decided to choose large teaching hospitals in expensive cities. My housing would be covered, and I thought there would be more to see and do in the places where people went on vacations. Why pay to stay in a metropolitan area when you could live there for free simply by working three or four days a week? It made perfect sense to me, and nurses were needed everywhere. When the time came to choose my first assignment, I had fourteen options to choose from. I started by going home to Chicago. It was February 1987, and I left the sunny skies of Texas behind as I drove into a blizzard.

The hardest part of leaving Galveston was saying goodbye to Louise, my roommate and dear friend. We met during hospital orientation in Galveston and became friends almost instantly. She worked as a recreational therapist in the psych hospital, and we shared a twisted sense of humor, tragic fashion choices, the ability to be amused by almost anything, and Midwestern values.

We both loved the *Man from Snowy River*, were the only female regulars at Monday Night Football, thought wearing Garfield pajamas in your twenties was acceptable, and saw nothing wrong with watching *Top Gun* weekly when it was in theaters. It was one of those rare friendships in which you knew you would always be accepted, protected, and supported. A true friend, she helped me move, wishing me luck in my new adventure and understanding it was something I needed to do. The future held endless possibilities, and I couldn't wait to get started.

Camp Nursing

My long-time habit of reading the help wanted ads every Sunday really paid off in the summer of 1987. I was finishing up a three month stint in a child psychiatry unit in downtown Chicago and had not decided where I wanted to go next. I was scanning the classifieds and enjoying a cup of coffee when a small ad caught my eye:

> *Camp for special needs children looking for a nurse. Camp begins in three weeks, and you will need to commit for eight weeks. If interested, please call.*

That was it. Just a few sentences in a page of larger ads, but it spoke to me. I called, and the next day drove one hour north to tour the camp and interview with the couple that had devoted their lives to this camp. They lived on the grounds with their two young sons, and it was clear from the moment we met that this was a match made in heaven. Everything clicked, and I felt at home. A few hours after I arrived, I happily accepted the position.

The camp sat on about 15 wooded acres, located right on Crooked Lake. Its mission was to provide a camp experience to children with physical disabilities. While the campers needed more time and assistance from the staff than children who did not have disabilities, they were at camp for the same reasons as any camper: fun, friendship, and a great experience.

The grounds included a recreation pavilion, a craft cabin, boat dock, fully-accessible pool, and the main lodge, which housed all the campers and counselors. It had a spacious dining room and comfortable living room. The lodge was a long, one-story building, and the campers were housed in six rooms that fed off a common hallway, each room accommodating six kids. The counselors stayed in a large room halfway down the hall, and the nurse's office, with a small attached bedroom, was at the beginning of the hallway. The layout was ideal for me because every camper and counselor would have to pass my door on the way to the living room, dining room, and front door. I could keep an eye on everyone very easily.

There would be four two-week sessions, each one having thirty-six campers. The first two sessions were the younger campers, aged eight to twelve. Those sessions were co-ed. The third session was teenage boys, and teenage girls comprised the final session. A great deal of planning went into each session, and spaces were given based on the individual needs of each camper. In each room of six, there were two campers who were considered "maximum help," meaning they needed a significant amount of assistance with toileting, feeding, dressing, and mobility. Two campers in the room were considered moderate help, needing a smaller degree of assistance. The last two campers in the room were called the runners—they were able to leave the room to get help if it was needed. As I learned during the first session, the term "runner" was a bit deceptive.

It was the third night of camp, and a full moon was streaming through my window. I was almost asleep when I heard a faint scratching sound that I couldn't quite place. I sat up and listened intently. Scratch, scratch, scratch...I opened my door, looking up and down the hall. Nothing. I started to close my door when something grabbed my ankle.

I jumped, tripped, and ended up on the floor, staring into the face of an equally startled nine-year-old boy. Joshua was the runner for room #3, and one of his roommates had a stomach ache. He had crawled down the hall and had been pressed against the wall so closely I hadn't seen him when I opened the door.

"Nurse Colleen, you jump high!"

I whispered, "And you are a very quiet crawler. I didn't hear you come down the hall, and I usually hear everything."

Joshua seemed pleased. "I can sneak around my house at night, and no one knows. I am a ninja crawler."

"You are indeed, Joshua. Shall we go check on your roommate?" I stood up, grabbed my bag, and followed him down the hall. He was really fast, and as he pulled himself back into his bed, he offered me a little free advice.

"Nurse Colleen? When you are looking around, don't forget to look down. Sometimes people are on the ground."

CHEESECAKE ON A STICK

Mealtime was a chaotic and always entertaining part of the day. Food prep was handled by Lisa, a college student majoring in Food Sciences. She tailored meals to an individual's allergies, religious requirements, and ability to chew. She had fifty plus meals promptly ready three times a day, and the food was really good. Once the food was on the table, we ate family style.

The first few meals each session were hilarious. It was fun to watch counselors try to learn what their campers needed. Some needed help cutting their food into bite-sized pieces, some needed help with adaptive devices, and some campers needed to be fed. Food ended up on the floor, on faces, on clothing, and often on the counselors. Every meal included laughter.

One morning, I was in the kitchen talking with Lisa about the allergies in the upcoming session when a van pulled up with food donations. The community was very supportive of the camp, and much of the food and supplies were donated. This delivery was all frozen food items. We helped unload vegetables, pizzas, waffles, fruit, and something I never knew existed: chocolate-covered cheesecake on a stick. Ten cases of chocolate dipped wedges-of-deliciousness.

Once the truck pulled away, Lisa looked at me, a smile tugging at the corner of her mouth. "Well, Colleen, I think it's clear what we have to do."

"We have a responsibility to our campers to do a little quality assurance."

She nodded her head. "What kind of chef would I be if I served something I hadn't tasted?"

"And what kind of nurse would I be if I didn't verify the ingredients? What if there were peanuts or if the sticks were a safety hazard? We owe it to the campers and counselors to make sure the food is safe." As I spoke, Lisa disappeared into the walk-in cooler, returning with two golden pouches. We peeled back the wrapping, revealing the wedge shaped chocolate covered goodies.

"To camp safety!" Lisa offered, holding the stick aloft.

"Safety first," I responded. "I would do anything for my campers."

It was delicious, passed through quality control with flying colors, and promised to be a huge hit with campers and counselors alike. It was terribly messy, melting quickly in the ninety degree heat we were experiencing that summer. No one complained about the mess, though, and we all agreed that it was well worth it. Life was simply better when it included chocolate-covered cheesecake on a stick.

THE FIRST QUESTION

I was in my office charting when I heard someone running down the hall. It was Shauna, out of breath and looking flustered.

"Nurse Colleen—something is wrong with Cindy and we need help. Please, come quick!" She turned and ran back down the hall. I was right behind her.

Cindy was a thin, fifteen-year-old with cerebral palsy. She did not talk but was able to communicate with sounds, expressions, and basic sign language. She had a beautiful smile, a great sense of humor, and was usually quite easy to understand. I found her stretched out on her bed, lying on her back and rocking in apparent discomfort.

"Cindy," I put a hand on her shoulder and made sure I had her attention so I could figure out what was wrong. "Are you in pain?"

Her eyes wide, she nodded yes emphatically.

"Is it a muscle cramp?"

"No," she signed.

"Are you sore from the way you were positioned in your wheel chair?"

"No."

"Is it your head?"

Cindy was rocking harder, her right arm extended, clearly signaling "No."

I was looking for any signs of injury: bruising, redness, a bug bite, splinter, sunburn, or blisters. I didn't see anything wrong with her, and she was looking at me as if to say, "You're the nurse, you should know what's wrong!"

I changed tactics, trying to localize the source of her pain. "Is it above your waist, Cindy?"

She groaned in frustration. "NO."

"It's below your waist, then, right? The problem is below your waist?"

She signed, "Yes" and grunted. I glanced down at her legs and froze, suddenly realizing what the problem was. How dense could I be? I met her gaze, and she knew that I knew. A smile spread across her face as I asked what should have been my first question, "Cindy, do you need to use the bathroom?"

Bingo. She gave a triumphant cry and started laughing. In the span of a few seconds, six campers, three counselors, and a nurse were laughing uncontrollably. It was too late to get her to the bathroom, and Cindy became one of several females in the room that evening who laughed so hard they wet their pants.

THE OFFICE

As camp nurse, my days started early and ended late. Some were busier than others, and I found that I wasn't always able to spend time I wanted to with Julie, the head counselor. Julie was a physical therapy student in graduate school and came from a tiny town in southwestern Nebraska. Greatly animated in front of the campers, she was quiet and reserved in private. This was her third year at camp, first as head counselor, and she went out of her way to help me acclimate to camp.

We tried to get together each morning to discuss the day's activities, but if a camper needed me, our time disappeared. We both understood the importance of knowing what the other was doing, so about a week into the first session, we decided to schedule office time each evening before we went to bed. Once I was satisfied that all of the campers were settled in for the night and she had checked in with the counselors, we went to the office, instructing the on-call staff to interrupt us only if "someone's hair was on fire, we needed to evacuate, or there was visible blood."

Our "office" was behind the lodge, right in the middle of the pool. It gave us privacy, a little relaxation, and exercise designed to offset the effects of cheesecake. We swam laps while discussing things that had happened during the day, changes we felt might be necessary for the next day, and any concerns we had. By the time we had completed our laps, we were on the same page and able to present a strong, united front.

It was a valuable lesson in the power of teamwork, and by the end of summer, Julie was one of my best friends. She gave me glimpses into life in a small Nebraska town, and I shared my hopes for the future. We both learned that if you took the time to really get to know the people around you, you might be rewarded with a wonderful friendship.

MEXICO

In September 1987, I had the opportunity to join my parents on a medical mission trip to Mexico. My parents, both social workers, were active in an organization called Healing the Children. Active is a bit of an understatement—my father would go on to be president of the non-profit, and both my parents served as leaders in the Illinois/Indiana chapter. It was a wonderful organization that provided medical screenings and treatment in other countries and arranged to bring children to the States for medical treatment not available in their home countries.

I was in the middle of an assignment in Stamford, Connecticut working on an adult psychiatry unit and had negotiated the time off when accepting the contract. I had chosen the location due to its proximity to New York and went into the city almost every weekend, trying to see as many of the sights as I could. One of the nurses I worked with introduced me to shopping on the streets of SoHo. My love for bargains was satisfied when I found a nice little grey suitcase with lots of storage compartments to take to Mexico. It was just $15, and I left for our trip feeling both stylish and thrifty.

The group I was invited to join was going to San Quintin, a town on the west coast of the central Baja California Peninsula, located several hours south of Tijuana. San Quintin had beautiful beaches and a level of poverty I had never before witnessed. We were there to screen children, perform minor surgical procedures, and treat minor illnesses. We were hosted by a local physician and worked out of the only hospital in the region. On the day of our arrival, we unpacked our supplies, set up exam stations, and became acquainted with the hospital layout.

On our second day in San Quintin, we were taken to one of the paper villages. I had never heard of a paper village and was completely unprepared for what I saw. It was a sprawling housing tract in which the walls of each home were comprised of Coca-Cola cartons, newspapers, and flattened cardboard boxes. No electricity and no indoor plumbing. The houses, huts to be more accurate, were tiny, maybe 10 feet by 10 feet. There were at least one hundred huts, and they were lined up in long rows with less than a foot of space between neighbors.

The bathrooms, which were communal, were up a small hill on one side of the village. The stalls had partial walls, no roofs, and afforded far less privacy than a port-a potty. You could look up the hill and see people's feet in the occupied stalls. At the base of the hill, there was a small pond, and women were washing both clothes and children in the water. Drinking water for the entire village was provided by a watering hole located in the center of the huts. The hole was about ten feet across and surrounded by a low stone wall. A bucket was lowered down into the hole with a rope and pulled up full of water.

It was the most primitive setting I had ever seen, and yet, there was a palpable sense of community and pride in the village. We were greeted with open arms, and the children grabbed our hands, pulling us towards their houses to show us where they lived. I was hugged and kissed, and more than a few of the girls wanted to play with my hair. In 1987, I was blonde, and my long, straight hair was a hit. I was, by far, the palest person in the paper village that day. We left with promises of seeing the children at the hospital during the week and took a long scenic route back into town.

Housing for our group was a bit of an issue, because there simply weren't enough hotel rooms to accommodate the entire team. As one of the younger members, I wasn't given a hotel room and was housed in the hospital. There was only one shower in the hospital, so each morning, I would walk across the street and use the shower at my parents' hotel. The water was only on at certain times of the day, so it was important to be on time.

My room in the hospital was used for childbirth, and the bed was an older model labor bed in which the bottom half was detachable. When it was time for a woman in labor to push, the bottom half was rolled away so the stirrups could be used. The bed had seen better days. The first time I turned over, the bottom half broke away and rolled a few feet across the room. I was unprepared for this and promptly fell to the floor. The second time it happened, I was able to grab the hand rails and hang on. It got to be pretty amusing. I tried tying the halves together, propping my feet in the stirrups, and sleeping with my head at the foot of the bed. I adapted and by the third night had learned to sleep in a tightly curled fetal position, keeping most of my body on the top half of the bed.

I was paired with Erik, a pediatrician from San Diego. We were assigned to pediatric medical screenings. Neither of us was fluent in Spanish, so we decided to split the human body in half. We agreed that I would handle "above the waist" questions, and Erik would be in charge of "below the waist" questions. Each of us would be responsible for half an exam. I memorized my questions and had a cheat sheet in my pocket if needed. It worked very well for us, and we became pretty proficient in completing exams efficiently.

Our first patient was a six-year-old boy named Jose who looked very healthy. Erik started the physical exam while I asked my half of the questions. My Spanish was far from perfect, but the boy's mother was very patient and helped me pronounce the words as I went through my list of questions.

How old is he?

Does he have any pain?

Where is the pain?

Any problems with his ears?

Any problems with his eyes? Itching, redness, drainage, or not seeing well?

Any problems with his nose? Itching, congestion, or runny nose?

Any problems with chewing or swallowing?

Any toothaches?

Does he sleep well?

Does he have a good appetite?

Does he have problems breathing?

Does he get tired easily?

Any problems with his neck, shoulders, arms, hands or fingers?

At this point, Erik took over, asking about digestion, bowel, bladder, and lower extremity issues. As happened with the vast majority of the children we examined, Jose was in excellent health and had no complaints. His mother simply wanted a doctor to examine him. When we told her he was a strong, healthy boy, she was so happy she cried, thanking us over and over again for helping her child.

Erik did not want to send her away empty-handed, so he ordered a bottle of Barnies, also known as Flintstone vitamins. It turned out that Barnies, Freds, Wilmas, and Bettys were the most prescribed medications that week. We gave them to each child we saw, and the parents had something to take home with them after waiting in long lines to have a child examined. I got quite good at saying, *"Debe tomar una pastilla cada mañana."* He should take one pill each morning.

We did see children with health issues, of course. Infected bug bites, rashes, cleft palates, dental abscesses, and poorly healed burns. The only source of heat in a paper village hut was an open fire in the middle of the floor. Sadly, children sometimes rolled into the flame while they were sleeping. Medical attention was not readily available, so the burns were left to heal on their own. When skin is burned, the surrounding skin begins to pull together, causing contractures. The resultant scarring can cause restrictions of movement around the injured area. With the kids we saw, it was most often an arm that was contracted and pulled tightly towards the chest wall. These kids were good candidates for trips to the US because surgical intervention could make a huge difference in their quality of life.

Minor surgeries were done during our stay in San Quintin. Dental procedures and wound care were the most common. Sterile technique is used for surgery, and the first time I heard an OR nurse say they needed someone to scrub in with a fly swatter I thought she was joking. She wasn't. The OR windows did not have glass and were open to the outside. Fly swatters were sterilized along with surgical equipment, and someone would stand at the table and swat the flies that came near the patient. Who knew?

We screened children for five days, seeing over two hundred in total. Some families walked for more than a day to get to the hospital, and we saw every single child that came. If nothing else, they left with toothpaste, a new toothbrush, and a bottle of Barnies. These children lived in abject poverty, but the vast majority of them were healthy and happy, and their parents just wanted to know they were doing a good job. It was a humbling and eye-opening experience, and I was happy to have shared it with my parents.

To this day, I can remember how to give instructions for taking antibiotics. *Es necesario tomar todas las pastillas. Uno por la mañana y el otro por la tarde, y por la noche.* It is necessary to take all of the pills. One in the morning, one in the afternoon, and one in the evening.

LOS ANGELES

I arrived in Los Angeles in January 1988, planning to work twelve-hour nights in a pediatric rehab unit. I ended up working the 3-11 shift on a general pediatric floor because the head nurse of the rehab unit decided that travel nurses were detrimental to staff morale. Hourly salaries for travelers were usually higher than those being paid to the staff nurses, and that sometimes led to resentment. Each unit handled travelers differently, and it was immediately clear pediatric rehab didn't want any.

In this case, it worked out really well for me because instead of working on a unit where I wasn't wanted, I was welcomed with open arms by 4West, a pediatric floor with twenty beds and outstanding nurses. There were six travel nurses working on the floor, so there was always someone to explore with.

Ruth, a nurse from Poughkeepsie, was all about the entertainment industry. We went to Universal Studios, walked the entire Hollywood Walk of Fame, and watched *Good Morning, Vietnam* and *Moonstruck* at Grauman's Chinese Theatre. It was pretty easy to get tickets to tapings of TV shows, and we were in the audience for *The Golden Girls, The Gary Shandling Show, The Tonight Show*, and a few completely forgettable pilots that never made it on the air.

Ginny was an arts buff, and we visited every museum we could find. The J. Paul Getty, which had free admission, became one of my favorites. Ginny had spent a few years in France and compared everything to the Louvre. It became a running joke, "So, is this bigger or smaller than the Louvre? Does the Louvre have nicer bathrooms? Are European artists featured in the Louvre?" Ginny and I visited the Queen Mary & Spruce Goose, drove to Santa Barbara for an art festival, and visited the La Brea Tar Pits.

Katie was the ultimate tourist, always carrying a travel guide in her enormous purse. She researched obscure attractions, knew every hole-in-the-wall restaurant worth visiting, and enjoyed coupons as much as I did. Katie and I discovered the joys of In-N-Out Burger, Pink's Hot Dogs, jambalaya at the Downtown LA Farmers Market, and, of course, Fat Burger. You couldn't visit LA without going to Fat Burger.

I had two roommates in LA, and we were a pretty good cross-section of why nurses chose to travel. I was traveling for the adventure, Autumn was traveling in order to save money to buy a house, and Kim had taken an assignment far from home in hopes of making her boyfriend miss her enough to propose. Adventure, financial gain, and short-term goals were the primary reasons nurses decided to become travelers. When you were lucky enough to work with nurses who had the same reasons, it was a blast.

It was a nice mix in LA, and I really enjoyed working with the staff nurses. The level of care was exceptional at Children's Hospital of Los Angeles, and I was a better nurse when I left. I saw as much of Los Angeles as I possibly could in thirteen weeks, but, looking back, what stands out more than anything else was the five-year-old who stole my heart.

BURT

I had just a few weeks left on my contract, and work was really busy. A strike by nurses at Los Angeles County's public hospitals had left us trying to care for more children than the unit could accommodate. There were a few kids on stretchers in the hallways, and everyone was scrambling to keep up with their assignment. Grace, the charge nurse, walked up to me with an apologetic smile on her face, and I knew my evening was about to get busier.

"I know you are running, Colleen, but we have a five-year-old coming up from the ER. He has 2nd and 3rd degree burns, and it's a bad situation. I am going to give your croup kid to Katie so you will have a little more time for the admission. I will help as much as I can."

"Okay. What kind of burns? Do we have any details?" Burn cases were tough, and caring for a child with burns was even tougher.

Grace's face, a picture of sadness, said it all. She shook her head, dropped her gaze, and gave me the short version. "Scalding water, bath tub, extensive burns below the waist, and splash burns on his arms, hands, and face. He's on heavy doses of morphine. Parents are being detained." She started to walk away but stopped long enough to voice a final thought. "How a parent can hurt their own flesh and blood is beyond me. I don't know if I could handle this admission, so thank you for doing it." Grace was six-months pregnant.

I met the stretcher as it came off the elevator, two staff in tow. The nurse walking beside the bed was holding a gauze-wrapped hand and saying, "You are such a brave boy, Burt. We are going to take good care of you, and it's gonna be okay." The ER nurse caught my eye, and the look on her face told me it was worse than I feared.

"I'm Colleen. I don't think we've met yet. Who is this you are bringing to me?" I stepped to the bedside and offered my hand to the nurse. We shook hands across the bed.

"Hi Colleen, I'm Letty, and this young man is Burt. Burt, meet Nurse Colleen. She is going to take very good care of you. We will get you all settled into your room and pretty soon it will be time for dinner. I will make sure you get that cheeseburger we talked about." She nodded towards the hallway and asked the ER attendant to stay with Burt for a minute. I followed her into the hall.

"I know the basics, Letty. That's all. Bathtub and hot water."

"Brace yourself. I don't care how many times you see it, you can't get used to it. If you do, it's time to get out of nursing, know what I mean? This one just makes me sick." Letty took a deep breath and filled me in on the details. Burt had wet his pants while taking a nap. His father had become angry and filled the tub with hot water, forcing his son into the tub to "think about what he had done." The water had reached the waistline of his jeans, and he sustained second degree burns from the waist down.

"So he was wearing jeans when he went into the tub?" I focused on details, not wanting to think about the big picture.

"Right. He must have had his legs bent, bunching up the denim behind his knees. The denim protected the skin there and it's much better than everything else. That's where you can put your hand when you change the dressings. It is really the only spot you can touch."

I sighed. "Poor kid. I'm not looking forward to hurting him." Dressing changes to burns were painful and involved pulling off layers of dying skin in order to allow healthy skin to grow. In order to help him, I was going to have to hurt him, and he had been hurt enough.

Letty finished briefing me, and I returned to the room to do my assessment and spend some time with Burt. He was a beautiful little boy with dark curly hair and impossibly long eyelashes. Freckles were splashed across his nose, and when I coaxed a small smile from him, a dimple appeared on his right cheek. He said "please" and "thank you," and my heart melted.

He was on pain medication and napped on and off for the first few hours of the shift. I watched him as he slept, taking in the extent of his bandages. He was wrapped in gauze from his waist to his toes, and his forearms and hands were covered as well. A few burns were visible on his neck and upper torso, most likely from splashing as he was pushed into the water. The extent of the dressing change was intimidating, and I decided to ask another nurse to help me so we could do both legs at once.

I didn't want to ask Grace, so I asked Ruth, the travel nurse I had become friends with. She had stopped by the room to ask if I needed anything, and I knew she had worked on a burn unit before. I gathered all of the supplies we would need, placing hers on one side of the bed and mine on the other. I pre-medicated Burt with a dose of morphine and told him we needed to take off his dressings and put on new ones that would be cool and less itchy. His mouth trembled a little, and he asked, very quietly, "Do we have to?"

"I'm sorry, Burt, but we have to. I will be just as fast as I can, and if you need to cry, that is fine. Crying is okay here, I promise."

"Okay, Nurse Colleen."

Ruth stood across the bed from me, and in unison, we started loosening tape and easing the gauze away from his skin. There is no easy way to pull dressing off burns, so when the time came to remove the inner layer of gauze, we planned to do it quickly, trying to limit the duration of his pain. His stoicism was breaking my heart. Every time a dressing was pulled, his face went white, but he didn't cry out or shed a tear.

We were ready to pull the dressing off his shins and ankle, and they were stuck pretty tight. I gathered the top of the dressing into my right hand and looked to see if Ruth was ready. She was, and the glitter of tears in her eyes brought tears to mine as well.

Unexpectedly, a gauze-covered hand reached up to wipe a tear trickling down my cheek. "It's okay, Nurse Colleen. I can take it." *He* was comforting *me*.

With a quick, "3, 2, 1," Ruth and I pulled the dressings, covered his skin with medication, and wrapped fresh gauze around his wounds. When we were done, I patted his shoulder and ruffled his hair.

"Thank you for helping us, Burt. I know that hurt, and I am sorry. You were very brave. Is there anything I can do to make you feel better before you go to sleep?"

"Could you read me a story? I like *Good Night, Moon.*"

"I think that can be arranged." Grace helped me find a copy, and Burt was fast asleep before we got to the final few pages. *Good night, stars. Good night, air. Good night, noises everywhere.*

I took care of Burt for the next three days, and each time I changed his dressings, he thanked me, asking "Will you be back tomorrow, Nurse Colleen? Will you take care of me tomorrow?"

My answer was, "Yes, I'll be back tomorrow, and I hope I can take care of you. I promise to read you a story before you go to sleep."

On the fifth day, I got off the elevator and headed for Burt's room, wanting to let him know I was there. He was gone, and a new child was in the room, crying and kicking at the nurse trying to start an IV. I hurried to the nursing station, thinking he must have been moved into a different room or to another unit. He was no longer a patient, though, and had been transferred to a different hospital that morning. The charge nurse from the day shift told me it was done for security reasons. Burt was gone, and I didn't get to say goodbye.

In nursing, closure is not a given. You often do not know what happens to your patients, don't have the opportunity to say goodbye, and sometimes come to work to find that the person you cared for the day before has died. It can leave you feeling hollow, unsettled, and sad. It is a part of the job that is difficult to accept but impossible to avoid. I hoped Burt didn't feel I had abandoned him. I certainly have not forgotten him.

SCRAPING BOTTOM

It is fair to say that not all assignments were created equal, and the two following Los Angeles were disappointing at best. I left Los Angeles in March 1988, heading towards New Orleans and planning to enjoy Jazz Fest while I was there. I had contracted with a large teaching hospital and was going to be working in the pediatric step-down unit. Step-down units were for kids who were too sick for a regular floor but did not need intensive care.

Some travel nurses flew to their assignments, but I always drove, wanting to have my car with me wherever I lived so I could explore more easily. I took a quick detour to Galveston, picking up my friend Louise so we could enjoy a weekend in New Orleans before I started my assignment. We started our drive when she got off work and reached New Orleans shortly before midnight. When we got to my assigned housing, we just laughed.

The sign in front of the building said, "Executive Housing," but there was nothing in its appearance to suggest that executives stayed there. It would never give an Extended Stay or All-Suite hotel any competition and seemed more like the type of place a transient might stay while trying to find housing.

"Well," Louise observed, "it is conveniently located right beside the highway off-ramp, making escape easy. And if you decide to open your windows, you are close enough to the highway to smell the diesel of passing trucks."

"Good point," I said, turning to the sad little pool. "And since they clearly haven't used chlorine for a while, perhaps it's been converted to a fishing hole."

"We can only hope. New Orleans is known for seafood."

"Plan B?" I suggested.

"If you are thinking of finding a hotel in which we might feel safe and consider using the shower, I would say, 'yes.' Plan B sounds like a very good plan."

Six hotels later, we were unable to find a room. There were several conventions in town and finding a hotel in New Orleans on a Friday night was more of a challenge than we expected. We ended up returning to the Executive Housing hotel. My housing had been arranged for me by my travel nurse agency, and all I had to do was pick up a key. We decided it was a better option than sleeping in my car, so we carried our things up to the second floor. When we let ourselves in, it was a very nice surprise. The one-bedroom unit was spacious, comfortably furnished, and spotless. It had a working kitchen and free cable, and the street noise wasn't bad at all.

The housing turned out to be the best part of my assignment. After a fun weekend with Louise that involved late hours, lots of jazz and a few too many cocktails, she returned to Texas, and I got ready for my assignment.

The reception the following day was chilly, and the charge nurse told me right away that they were not thrilled that "outsiders" were being brought in. I was the only travel nurse working in pediatrics, and I had a feeling it was going to be a lonely stay. I asked about the unit rules, what I was and was not allowed to do as an RN, and got to work. The charge nurse watched me start an IV on a teenager with cellulitis and told me I was taping the IV incorrectly. I asked her to show me the way they wanted IVs secured, and learned a seventh "correct" way to tape an IV.

I actually liked the way they taped IVs, and it reminded me that even when an assignment wasn't great, I could still learn a lot. Most hospitals had a firm opinion on the "right" way of doing things, and travelers collected techniques as they passed through. It gave us tremendous flexibility and adaptability. It is nice to know a dozen ways to accomplish the same task, and I tried to adapt to each unit I worked in.

I had my limits, though, and reached them at 6 am during my first overnight shift. It had been a hectic night, and I was trying to get my charting done before the day shift arrived. I was finishing up with the second of four charts when the residents and medical students walked down the hall, arriving at the nursing station. Two of my coworkers left the station immediately, but I didn't give it much thought. I felt someone staring at me, and when I looked up from my chart, I noticed I was the only nurse still in the nursing station.

"Good morning," I began, speaking to the third year resident who was staring at me. "Can I help you with something? Do you need one of these charts?"

He studied me for a minute before answering, "I'd like to sit down and am wondering why you are still here."

"In the nursing station? Why wouldn't I be here?"

"You should vacate your chair when a physician approaches. That's the way it's done here, so you're in my seat."

I laughed. He didn't, and when the charge nurse told me I needed to apologize, I realized I would not be staying for Jazz Fest. There were some policies I simply was not willing to adapt to, and it was time to move on. I was happy to leave and am quite sure they were glad to see me go.

The very next day, I handed in the keys to my executive housing and hit the road. It hadn't taken long to pack my car because my things only fit one way. I packed the car exactly the same way each time, using two milk crates, a garment bag, three suitcases, half a dozen tote bags, a small hanging file container, and, of course, my coffee pot. It sat right behind me in a place of honor, the last thing loaded and the first taken out of the car. Priorities.

The front seat held a six-can cooler stocked with Fresca and Diet Vernors, a Tupperware container full of snacks, an overnight bag, and my beloved cassette tape collection. I sang my way from city to city, especially enjoying the mixed tapes I'd painstakingly created. "Metal Mix" and "Men Are Pigs" were my favorites.

I had traveling down to a science. I left every morning at 7 am, and covered between 650-750 miles a day. I checked into a hotel by 7:15 pm, picked up dinner, and had a picnic on my bed while watching whatever HBO movie began at 8:00 pm. In the late 1980s, HBO was a luxury, and I chose hotels that offered a free movie. There was only one HBO channel, so the choice was made as soon as you turned the TV on. I went to sleep when it ended, and repeated the process each day until I arrived in my new city.

Three days and two movies later, I arrived on Long Island, New York, where I was to begin an eight-week assignment in a pediatric step-down unit, working twelve-hour nights.

THE FAT FARM

"What do you mean there isn't a step-down unit? I was hired to work twelve-hour nights in pedi step-down." I was sitting across the desk from the nurse recruiter, filling out paperwork and picking up the keys to my housing, which was being provided by the hospital. This wasn't the start I was hoping for.

She was unfazed, shrugging her shoulders. "There must have been some confusion. I have you down for eight hours nights on the general pediatric floor."

"Then, we have a bit of a problem," I observed. "I don't work eight hour shifts and was planning on working step-down. How can I be hired for a unit that doesn't exist, working twelve-hour shifts you don't offer? That's a pretty big misunderstanding." I had heard from other travel nurses that sometimes you were given misleading information and now understood what they meant.

"It's not a problem. We're happy to let you work on the peds floor."

"Not an option for me. I am not going to work eight hour nights." It was much harder to explore an area when you were working five nights a week, and I was an hour away from New York City. If I worked twelve-hour shifts, I would have 3-4 days off each week to be a tourist, and since I had chosen this assignment because I wanted to spend more time in New York City, I wasn't going to negotiate shifts.

"Well…I guess we could put you in neonatal ICU. They work twelve hour shifts there."

"Do they have a grower's room?" When premature infants were healthy enough to leave neonatal ICU but not big enough to go home yet, they were placed in the grower's room, a unit adjacent to the NICU where they basically gained weight until they reached their goal for discharge. Depending on the hospital, 4 ½ to 5 pounds was the target weight.

"Of course. Why don't I give the head nurse a call, and you can go meet her."

I met the head nurse of the NICU and took a tour of their large and very busy unit. They were understaffed, and she told me I would be a welcome addition. I wasn't a neonatal nurse, but she assured me that I would be placed only in the grower's room and that "If you can feed, burp, and change a baby, you will be just fine." It sounded good to me, so I accepted the position, unloaded my car, and started that evening.

I changed into the turquoise scrubs worn by the NICU nurses and stepped into the grower's room. The room was about 20 feet by 30 feet, and the walls were lined with tiny cribs and isolettes (enclosed cribs), each one with a small table beside it. There were no windows, and the lighting was dim. In the center of the room, there were five rocking chairs, all vacant. I was alone with fifteen infants, and many of them were crying.

A voice spoke softly into my ear, close enough to startle me. "You must be Colleen. Welcome to the Fat Farm! I'm Jean, and I'm really glad you're here." I turned around and found myself face-to-face with a forty-something woman carrying a large load of blankets, diapers, and wipes. I took the blankets out of her arms and followed her to the supply cart at the far end of the room. Once everything was put away, she extended a hand to shake mine, and gave me a warm, sincere smile. I smiled back, relieved.

"I'm glad to be here, Jean. Will it be just the two of us?"

"Honey, until I found out you were coming, it was looking like it would be just the one of me. We are really short-staffed, and when we fill up, it gets crazy." She pointed to the cribs. "When we are full, we have to line the cribs back to back to make room for all the babies. We're supposed to hold sixteen, but most of the time we have 20-24."

"And the two of us can handle 24 babies?" I had my doubts.

"Here's how it works. I have a system that, if I say so myself, is just about perfect." She smiled. "Babies are fed either every three or every four hours. As soon as we get here, we make sure we know who is who and put an empty bottle on top of every three-hour eater. We feed them first, starting with whoever is awake or, more likely, who is screaming the loudest. Once all the three hour bottles are gone, we start on the four-hour eaters. Once they are done, we start over. We do it over and over again until it's time to go home. Feed them, burp them, change them, and move on. Any questions?"

I liked her and appreciated her attitude. "Just show me where I chart, where to find their schedule, and which rocker is mine."

"Colleen, you can have any rocker my backside isn't parked in. Let's get to work."

Jean and I worked very well together, and the night went exactly as she said it would. Feed, burp, change, and move on. Repeat until it is time to go home. The first night I repeated the process twenty-eight times. The night flew by, and I was happy to learn that my schedule would mirror Jean's. I worked with her every single shift, and we became friends, one five-minute conversation at a time.

I learned how to burp even the most resistant baby and could change a diaper in about ten seconds. Jean showed me how to calm a drug-addicted baby, telling me in her blunt way that "If you can learn to calm a cocaine baby, you can rule the world." We had a few alcohol and drug addicted babies, lots of preemies needing to fatten up so they could go home, and an occasional baby sent from the regular nursery because they needed antibiotics or extra monitoring.

Jean and I rocked as we fed the babies, talking about family, men, friends, men, vacations, men, and whatever else came up. Over the course of my eight weeks on Long Island, I became a much better neonatal nurse and a world-class burper. Plus, I found a friend in a place I never would have chosen to be. Sometimes things just work out, and if I hadn't already made plans for the summer, I would have stayed awhile longer.

I hugged Jean goodbye, thanking her for welcoming me to the fat farm and making it such a good experience. I turned in my keys, loaded my car, and drove west. It was time to go back to camp.

PERSPIRING PETE

The week before camp started was an exercise in controlled chaos. Counselors met for the first time, the rooms were set up, the rec hall and crafts cottage prepared, and we all got to know each other a little better. We also had several training sessions, and I gave talks on basic first aid, allergies, safety during mealtimes, and anything about the individual campers I thought we should cover. I made sure to talk about heat stroke and heat exhaustion because camp was not air conditioned and we were in the midst of a brutal heat wave.

I tried to come up with little sayings or verbal cues that would help the staff remember the things we had talked about. I was particularly pleased with my poem about heat related disorders: *Perspiring Pete says sweat is sweet, but if you're hot, dry and red, look out kids, you'll be dead.* That one seemed to stick.

It was much easier getting my office ready because I knew what I was doing this time around. It can be difficult to go into an office set up by someone else, and that had been the case the summer before. I had struggled to make sense of the choices made by the nurse who came before me. This year, the nurse before me was *me*, so everything seemed logical and exactly where it should be. Most nurses are organized, but pediatric and neonatal nurses are obsessive about it. I fit into that category very easily and found organization to be relaxing.

Disorganization, on the other hand, was a sure sign that I was stressed. If I couldn't find my pens and lost track of what I was doing, it was time to take a deep breath and regroup. At camp I never lost my pens because I was too busy to be stressed. It was an entertaining and very rewarding busy that I absolutely loved.

A really fun part of preparing for the campers was decorating the lodge. Each summer had a different theme, and that year, we decorated with the animals of Sandra Boynton. Her cows, cats, rabbits, ducks, and chickens covered the walls.

Julie was back as head counselor and stopped by my office with the all-important question. "So, Colleen, what kind of animal do you want to be? They are getting ready to make a sign for your door, so you get to pick."

I didn't have to give it much thought. "I think I would like to be a pig."

"Pig? Really? You want a pig that says 'Colleen' on your door?"

"Not just any pig, Julie. I would like a pig with a crown. It would be perfect, and the kids will love it." It seemed like a good idea, a cute Boynton pig wearing a crown.

Julie looked dubious. "A big pink pig with a crown. Hmmm... sometimes I wonder about you." She laughed as she turned away, and a few moments later I heard her announce to the counselors, "Colleen wants a pig with a crown." And that's exactly what I got. A two-foot tall pig wearing a gold crown that said, "Nurse Colleen." No one was going to miss my door, and I loved it.

WRESTLING ALLIGATORS

Summer is supposed to be hot, but the summer of 1988 was *really* hot. Illinois was in a record-setting drought, and during the course of the summer, the temperatures exceeded 100 degrees seven times. All seven times, camp was in session. Activities had to be changed to protect both campers and counselors from heat exhaustion, dehydration, and heat stroke.

Every camper and counselor carried water bottles, and we equipped everyone with squirt guns or spray bottles. I called random "Hose down your counselor" and "Water your camper" drills, and everyone was drenched. I played waitress, delivering Dixie cups of juice and water, and we spent a great deal of time in the pool. Our efforts succeeded, and in spite of the heat, no one had a heat-related illness that summer.

On a particularly sweltering Friday afternoon, we had a pool party, and everyone was either in the water, sitting on the edge, or sitting in a chair as close to the edge as we could get it. Hoses, wet towels, sponges and buckets of water were used to keep people comfortable. Always looking for new and different activities, someone came up with the idea of wrestling inflatable pool floats. The campers would choose a staff member, and the chosen one would dive into the pool and put on a show, trying to wrestle the float into submission. I was watching the spectacle through my office window as I got evening meds ready, and it was hilarious.

The last float to be launched was the alligator, a six-foot beast that rose a good foot above the water level. I was wondering who would be next when I heard a faint voice call out, "Where's Nurse Colleen?"

"Nurse Colleen! Nurse Colleen! Nurse Colleen!" The voices grew louder, and Julie rapped on my window from outside. "I believe you have been chosen. Lock up and give us a show." How could I turn down such a request? I locked my office and jogged out, pumping my fists in the air, ready to defeat my opponent.

The campers cheered, and the staff laughed. I dove in, resurfacing right in front of the alligator's snout. They cheered, and I poked him in the eye. They cheered louder, and I grabbed him by the tail, flipping him onto his back. I started climbing onto him, planning to declare victory when I discovered it was harder than it looked to mount an inflatable alligator in the deep end. Halfway up, it tilted, and we both flipped over. The campers went wild, thinking it was part of the show.

I was successful on my 4th or 5th attempt, riding the gator in the deep end, my hands clasped above my head in triumph. I looked around the pool, soaking it in. Counselors were clapping, and my campers were cheering, laughing, and smiling. It just doesn't get any better than that.

FAREWELL TO THE PIG

Camp came to an exhausting end with tearful goodbyes, promises to stay in touch, and many, many hugs. A few hours after the last camper was picked up, I was packed up and ready to head home, scheduled to fly to Germany the next morning. I had scheduled four weeks in Europe before heading to my next assignment.

Leaving meant I was going to miss the staff banquet, which would be held later that evening. Camp tended to create close friendships and saying goodbye wasn't easy. I knew there would be more than a few tears shed that evening and that many of the counselors would opt to stay another night. Julie walked me to my car, and we lingered for a few minutes, postponing the inevitable.

"Take pictures for me tonight, okay?"

"Of course," she said, "and don't forget to visit me next time you pass through Nebraska. The family would love to meet you."

"I'll try. You know, there is one thing that would entice me there for sure."

She made a good guess, "Cheesecake-on-a-stick?"

"Tempting, but I was thinking of blow-drying a cow." During one of our late night swims, she had told me about blow-drying her cow before a 4H competition in order to make its coat shinier. I wanted to see this in person.

"If you come, we will definitely blow-dry a cow."

"Deal. I don't know when, but I'll make it to Nebraska."

We hugged, knowing it was going to be our last summer at camp. She would be starting clinical rotations for her masters in physical therapy, and I had no idea where I might be the following summer. Two summers of great memories would be the extent of our time together.

When I got back from Germany four weeks later, there was a package waiting for me at my parents' house. As promised, Julie had taken pictures at the staff banquet. There was a group shot, with the counselors lined up three deep. Next to Julie, front row and center, was the two-foot-tall pig with a crown that had spent the summer on my office door. Nurse Colleen had made it after all.

BOSTON, 1988

I had heard about the beauty of New England in the fall, so when I had the chance to work in a child psych unit in Boston I took it, arriving in September as the leaves were just starting to change. I was housed in Quincy, a town a few minutes outside of town and a short commute to my hospital. The mass transit system, called the "T," was easy to navigate, and I took the Green line. It was my first time using mass transit, and I was grateful to avoid driving in Boston, which seemed to be in a perpetual state of construction.

I was the only travel nurse working in child psych, and the reception was mixed. The sense of cohesion I had felt in Galveston was not present, and there was a clear discrepancy in philosophies on how to interact with the kids. There is a saying among healthcare providers that many people go into psychiatry/psychology because they have psych issues themselves, and that seemed to apply to some of my coworkers. There was a lot of "processing" of our feelings taking place in the nursing station when I felt time would be better spent with our kids. I found the day shift to be a difficult mix of staff personalities and was more than willing to change to the 3-11 shift when asked.

Much better. I connected almost immediately with Sam, a nurse from Connecticut who had worked in other units and saw the staff dynamics I was struggling with. Sam was blessed with a calming presence that the kids gravitated to, and she instinctively knew when to step back and when to step in. We shared a twisted sense of humor and were soon spending time together outside of work. I appreciated having someone to do things with, and Boston had a lot to offer.

Sam lived in the North End, the center of Boston's Italian population. Her apartment was right off the Freedom Trail, a 2 ½ mile trail that wound through downtown, passing many of the city's historic landmarks. It started at the visitor information center in Boston Common and ended at the USS Constitution in

Charlestown. I walked the trail several times, always finding something new.

Sam and I had long conversations at Caffe Vittoria, an Italian café that had been in operation since 1929. Their cappuccino was outstanding, and we put a pretty good dent in their pastry menu, trying something new each time we went. As with every city I visited, one place stood out as a favorite. Here, it was Caffe Vittoria, hands down.

It always struck me as odd that travel nurses seemed to know more about hidden gems than the locals did. Maybe it was because we knew we had such a short time to see what the area had to offer, or maybe it was due to the fact that we had limited responsibilities outside of work. Whatever the reason, if you wanted to know where to go, you asked another traveler. While I was the only one in child psych, there were several travel nurses in my apartment building, and they sent me on great day trips.

Polly's Pancake Parlor in Sugar Hill, New Hampshire served the best pancakes I ever tasted. A gorgeous 2 ½ hour drive from my apartment, it was just twenty minutes from Franconia Notch State Park, home of the famous Old Man of the Mountain. If you combined the two destinations, you could hike off the pancakes before returning to Boston.

I took a solo trip to Maine after being told I "had to go to Moody's Diner" for muffins and a stay in one of their cabins. It was a beautiful drive, and the muffins were as good as I had been told. I stayed the night in one of the small cabins behind the diner, and it was like walking back in time. The phone had rotary dial, the TV was black & white, and the heater was a plug-in unit that looked to be about a hundred years old. I curled up into the worn but very comfortable armchair and read a book cover to cover. It was a lovely weekend.

Julie came to visit me, as did my parents and my sister Betsy. I took all of them to the Bull and Finch Pub, where exterior shots for the TV show *Cheers* were filmed. The bartender's name was Sam (or so he said), and it was always fun to eat there. Trips to Cape Cod,

Salem, Providence, RI and Mystic, CT filled my weekends. When Sam and I went to see Boston Ballet's *Swan Lake* at The Boston Opera House, it was the first and only time I ever saw a ballerina get dropped.

Almost all my touring took place on the weekends because I was working at least five days a week and pulling double shifts when needed. The unit stayed full, and staffing was inadequate. It was hard to turn down an additional shift when you knew what it would mean to the staff you were leaving. On a chaotic Thursday, when I was fourteen hours into a sixteen-hour double, I had the most frightening experience of my nursing career.

TRAPPED

His name was Dan, and he was an angry seventeen-year-old in the midst of a psychotic break. Standing 6'2" and topping the scales in excess of 250 pounds, he was an imposing presence, and we had been double teaming him since his arrival two days earlier. His medications had been ineffective, so his psychiatrist had admitted him so one medication could be withdrawn while a different anti-psychotic was begun. It was called "washing out," meaning you let one medication clear before starting over in hopes of finding a better combination of drugs. What that meant to us was that he had very little medication in his body and would be likely to display whatever behaviors came with his psychosis. It was not fun for him or for us.

He clearly had auditory hallucinations and had conversations with the voices he was hearing. He kept to himself for the most part, refusing to participate in activities, groups, and individual counseling sessions. I caught him staring at me several times, and his malevolent expression made me really uncomfortable. There was an open hostility that seemed to be aimed in my direction.

A younger patient told the unit secretary that Dan had said something about "stabbing the demon," and when she called me into the hall to tell me this, I decided to do a room check to make sure we hadn't missed anything that could be used as a weapon. I let the other nurse know what I was doing and headed down the hall to Dan's room. For reasons, I will never understand, she told Dan what I was doing, and with a bellow of rage, he launched himself down the hall.

He entered his room, furious, and I was trapped. He stood between me and the door, the hostility I had seen over the past few days boiling over. His face contorted, and I felt a cold wave of fear. He was a foot taller, a hundred pounds heavier, and not in any state in which I could negotiate with him. I was absolutely still, trying not to appear threatening in any way.

"You're a demon." It wasn't a question; it was a statement. "Can't fool me. I know what you are."

He wanted to stab the demon, I thought. Where were the other staff members? Was anyone going to help me? I looked down, not wanting to engage him, hoping his anger would subside. Thoughts raced through my mind as I tried to come up with a strategy or response that wouldn't make it worse. I thought back to Galveston and the stories I had heard from the adult psych nurses, and the thought "use whatever power they give you" came to mind. I was on my own, so I gambled.

"Do you know my name? Or what I am capable of?" I met his gaze, raised my chin, and smiled the way Voodoo Mary had years before when she frightened me. I also prayed.

"No, ma'am." He dropped his gaze and backed out of his room. I found the plastic knives hidden under his mattress, made my way to the nurse's station, and stayed there until I stopped shaking. Once I got home, I fell apart, crying myself to sleep.

I had two weeks left in Boston, and the only time I felt safe on that unit was when I was working with Sam. I decided that short-term assignments in child psych were not a good idea because it was hard to develop trust among staff members quickly. This was going to be the last child psych unit I would work in.

I said my goodbyes, happy that I was leaving with a friendship that would continue. Sam sent me on my way in style, writing a hilarious poem.

Ode to a Goddess
There once was this bitchin' psych nurse named Colleen
She was a HOT thing; she was a nursing queen!
She came a flyin' in from distant cities
To be therapeutic with majorly whacked out kiddies,
Now she's traveling on from this hub town to the San Fran scene

Not too surprisingly, it was the first and only ode ever written about me.

STARTING THE YEAR WITH A BANG

January 1, 1989 found me in Orleans, Nebraska. I was on my way to San Francisco, and stopped to visit Julie. After two summers at camp, I had heard so much about her hometown that I just had to see it. Nebraska was playing Miami in the Sugar Bowl that evening, and every house in the small town was festooned in Nebraska's crimson and cream. As soon as I arrived, her brother Matt handed me a sweatshirt so I would fit in.

"We'll need to head out now," Matt said. "Word on the street is you want to blow-dry a cow. We have lots of cows to choose from, but we have to be home before kick-off. Everything stops when the game begins."

"Understood. Look out, cows, here I come." Julie and I squished into the front seat of Matt's pickup and headed out to their farm, where dozens of cows were blissfully unaware of my mission. They idly watched us as we pulled in, a few wandering up to the truck to look into the bed.

Julie explained, "They're hoping we have hay in the back. It will be easier if we grab one already near the barn." We drove to the barn, and I met Lucy, a brown and white heifer who looked like she could use a little TLC. Julie showed me the dryer, which looked a lot like a car wash vacuum. It was basically a long gray hose attached to a heater.

Lucy stood patiently as I learned the steps of effectively blow-drying a cow. I wet down her coat with a big, sloppy sponge, and then brushed against the grain, using the blow dryer close to her skin. When her coat was almost completely dry, I brushed the hair back into place, and *voilà,* it was shiny and more voluminous. I had fun, Matt and Julie had a good laugh, and I think Lucy was pleased.

Sadly, Nebraska did not fare well in the Sugar Bowl, losing 23-3. But it was fun to watch it with Julie's family, who welcomed me into their home and went out of their way to make my short visit memorable. As the football party wound down, her uncle offered to take us out for a buggy ride the following morning, and although I had a long drive ahead of me, I wasn't going to turn down an offer like that.

At 7:30 am, Julie and I were picked up in an open-air carriage pulled by two beautiful black horses. It was a clear, crisp, and very chilly day. Nebraska isn't known for its balmy January temperatures, and we huddled under blankets, enjoying the scenery and her uncle's non-stop stream of stories.

"If you get really cold, the heater's under the seat," he said. "Just reach under and grab it. No sense freezing to death."

Julie smiled, and I immediately reached under the seat, grabbing the only thing I found. It was a bottle of peppermint schnapps, a heat source I had never considered.

"No sense in freezing to death," Julie said, and who was I to disagree? Turns out, it worked. The rest of our buggy ride was a little more toasty.

SAN FRANCISCO, 1989

Opportunities arise when you least expect them, and when I was discussing available assignments with Keri, my recruiter, she told me an unusual contract was available in San Francisco. There was a hospital so short on pediatric ICU nurses that they had decided to offer travel nurses a thirty-day orientation in exchange for a nine-month commitment. So if I agreed to live (for free) in San Francisco for ten months total, I would be able to expand my nursing skills and become a better nurse. This particular peds ICU was well-known for a busy and very successful cardiac program, and I was thrilled to take advantage of this offer.

It was one of the best decisions I ever made. The nurses in the unit were great and the level of care exceptional. My preceptor had been a peds ICU nurse for eight years and knew exactly what she was doing. She took me under her wing, and I soaked up everything I could during my thirty-day training. I loved working with the open-heart kids and found that cardiac nursing came pretty easily to me. It made sense, and the logic was appealing.

In addition to being really good nurses, the staff in PICU were also very fun. The travel nurses were absorbed into the unit as if we were part of the family, and we encouraged the staff nurses to join us on our adventures. There were 8-10 travel nurses at any given time, so there was always someone to explore with.

I quickly became close with Ann, a travel nurse from North Carolina. It cracked me up that she always introduced herself by saying "I'm Ann from Raleigh, North Carolina." She had a great laugh, and we had similar interests. We traveled to Monterey, Pacific Grove, and Carmel. We visited most of the museums in San Francisco and enjoyed many Irish Coffees at Buena Vista, a popular tourist destination near Fisherman's Wharf.

Peggy, one of the staff nurses, took it upon herself to make sure we tried the restaurants only the locals knew about. Groups of us met regularly at Tien Fu on the corner of 21st & Noriega. As Peggy had promised, it had the best garlic chicken on the planet. We visited hidden restaurants in Chinatown, had fantastic Italian in the North Beach neighborhood, and agreed the Cliff House had the best omelets. We were introduced to 99-cent Hot White Russians at The Patio Café on Castro Street.

I went hot air ballooning over Napa Valley, visited dozens of wineries, and went to all of the usual tourist destinations San Francisco was famous for. It was a beautiful city, and there was always something to do. I liked my housing, the hospital, and the people I worked with, and I was surrounded by travel nurses I considered friends. It was a great situation.

In this beautiful city by the bay, amidst laughter, friendship, and adventure, I learned about death. Fighting it, accepting it, and embracing it.

LUKE

When I arrived in the pediatric intensive care unit shortly before 7 am, Luke's parents were waiting for me. Over the course of several months, we had spent many, many hours together and had developed a close bond. As soon as I saw their faces, I knew the decision had been made.

I had been taking care of their son for more than three months. In spite of being critically ill, he displayed a spunky little personality. He liked having his feet rubbed, would grab my stethoscope as I leaned over to listen to his heart and lungs, and when he was uncomfortable, his forehead would furrow into three distinct lines. I had spent hundreds of hours caring for him and had become quite attached.

He had undergone heart surgery when he was only three days old, and things had not gone well. In the first few months of his life, Luke had four surgeries and more procedures than I could count. The physicians in this unit were both progressive and open-minded, and when Western Medicine appeared to be failing, they were more than willing to try the Eastern Medicine Luke's parents requested. Salves and medicinal teas were flown in from family members in China and given in hopes of improvement. Unfortunately, Luke was succumbing to a fungal infection that did not respond to any of the treatments we had tried.

Luke's parents had slowly come to accept that they would not be taking their son home. It was one of those things you could see in the eyes, the eyes of every parent having to come to the terrible realization that they would be losing a child. On this particular morning, their eyes were simply sad.

"Nurse Colleen. Good morning." Luke's father bowed slightly as he greeted me.

"Good morning, Joe." My Cantonese was non-existent, and when I struggled to master the correct pronunciation of his name, Luke's father had told me to call him Joe.

"We are ready." His words hung in the air as the three of us looked at each other.

I nodded. "OK. Would you like me to get Dr. Carey, or do you want to sit with him for a few minutes?"

"You'll be with us, right?"

"Of course. I will be with you for as long as you want me to be. Dr. Carey will come in, make sure that you are comfortable with your decision, and then I'll hand him to you so you can hold him."

I paused, hesitating to remind them of the hardest part. "Like we talked about, it could be a few seconds, a few minutes, or a few hours. Each child is different."

Luke's parents looked at each other, clasped hands, and walked over to the crib where their son was lying. They looked at him, looked at me, and bowed their heads.

"We are ready, Colleen. "

I left Luke's room, closing the door softly, scanning the unit for the crowd of people that represented early morning rounds. Every morning the residents, fellows, and attending physician made the rounds of every bed in the pediatric intensive care unit. They discussed the events of the previous twenty-four hours and formulated the plan of care for the coming day. I saw them crowded around bed space #2. Luke was in bed #9, and I decided we couldn't wait for seven more beds.

Dr. Carey saw me coming. A few days earlier, I had stood next to him as he gave Luke's parents the news that treatment options had been exhausted, and their son's prognosis was bleak. He delivered this heartbreaking message with the honest compassion that endeared him to staff and families alike. He was, and would be, one of the finest physicians I was fortunate enough to cross paths with.

He raised an eyebrow, asking me if they were ready. I nodded, and he excused himself from the group. He sat down to talk with Joe and Liu, reviewing everything that had been tried and saying that he did not believe Luke could survive without the ventilator and medications supporting his vital signs. He was calm, quiet, and direct.

There were a few moments of silence as Dr. Carey let the information settle in the room. "Do you have any questions?"

Joe answered. "No. We understand."

"Do you want more time to think about this?"

"No. We are ready."

"Okay. I will turn off the ventilator, remove the breathing tube, and let you hold him. Colleen, will you help me?"

I removed the EKG pads, oxygen saturation monitor, and all the IVs except for one, which was kept in case pain medications were needed. I wrapped him up in blankets, loosened the tape holding the breathing tube in place, and signaled I was ready. Dr. Carey turned off the ventilator and pulled out the breathing tube. I wiped Luke's face and placed him in Liu's arms. Joe was sitting beside her, one arm wrapped tightly around her shoulders and the other arm placed gently across Luke's legs.

Luke lived for over an hour, his skin turning duskier and his breathing more ragged with each passing minute. During a period of calm, I saw hope cross their faces and prayed that Luke wouldn't struggle much longer. Hope can be cruel when death is imminent.

I was in the room, kneeling in front of Liu, when Luke died. It had been seventy-two minutes since he was taken off life support. He took a small breath and then did not take another. After waiting a few minutes that seemed to last hours, I listened for Luke's heartbeat one last time. Silence.

Dr. Carey came in to officially pronounce death. Joe shook his hand and thanked him for trying to save his son. As Dr. Carey left the room, I asked Liu and Joe if they would like me to give them some time alone. Liu kissed Luke's tiny hand and placed his body into my waiting arms. "We will leave him to you, Colleen. He is gone, and you must do what you need to do."

I bathed Luke's bruised and swollen body, trying to remove the stickiness of the tape I had applied to secure his IVs, breathing tube, chest tubes, and drains. I realized I had never seen his face without tape on it and had never picked him up without having to organize the spaghetti of lines that accompanied intensive care. As I cleaned his tiny hands, I remembered how tightly he had grasped my fingers the first time I bathed him. I wished he would squeeze my hand one more time.

The charge nurse entered the room, bringing the requisite paperwork and a body bag. "Colleen, have you done a morgue packet here before?"

"No, he's my first." I didn't elaborate. I had cared for children that died, but Luke was the first child I helped take off life support, the first child I handed to a mother so she could hold him as he died, and the first child I ever prepared for the morgue.

"Well, it's pretty straight forward. Just complete the form, make sure he has his ID bands on, use the bag, and deliver him to the morgue. You will have to sign the logbook when you get there, and that's pretty much it. There is a stretcher outside the door you can use if you want to."

"The morgue is in the basement, right?"

"Isn't it always? You need anything, or are you okay?"

"I'm all set. I'll just be a few minutes more—I know we need to turn the room." It was a very busy day, and there were kids in the ER waiting for beds to become available.

I opened the body bag, a one-size-fits-all plastic wrap that dwarfed Luke's body. I zipped him into its cold embrace and folded the bag several times to make it close to the appropriate size. I decided I would carry him to the morgue instead of letting him be swallowed up on an adult sized stretcher.

I wrapped a baby blanket around the bag and took him in my arms. The paperwork was held against me, between our bodies. As I walked out of his room, the housekeeper held the door for me before pushing her cart through. While I delivered Luke to the morgue, his room would be readied for the next child.

I left the unit and headed down the hall to the service elevator. I had a bit of a wait, and right as the doors slid open, I felt their presence behind me. Cradling their child's body against my chest, I turned to face them. Luke's parents, eyes swollen and red, asked me a silent question. *Please? Can we join you?*

The public was not supposed to use these elevators, but I was not about to deny them these last few moments as a family. I nodded, and they joined me in the oversized space. I pushed "B" and stood between them, Liu at my right shoulder and Joe at my left. We rode seven floors down in absolute silence, and as we neared the basement, I felt tears welling in my eyes. Liu put her hand on my shoulder, and a tear coursed down my cheek.

They did not try to go any further, staying on the elevator as I exited. I turned to look at them one last time, and they both bowed, hands pressed together as if in prayer. I shifted my grasp, placing my right hand on Luke's back so it would be over my heart. I waited for the doors to close before turning away.

My vision was blurred with tears, but I made it to the right door and rang the bell. The door was opened by a middle-aged woman in green scrubs. Her name badge said LaVerne.

"You got a little one for me today. Bless his little... her little??" Her voice trailed off.

"His. His name is Luke." I stood still, not knowing where she wanted me to go.

"Come this way, child. You care for him long?" She indicated a stainless steel table and gently took Luke from my arms, placing him onto the table and checking the paperwork.

"Since he was three days old, about three months now. Very nice family. Beautiful little boy. Sad to say goodbye."

LaVerne nodded, "You always feel it, don't you? I've seen so many children come through these doors in the past twenty years, and it's never easy. How many times have you made this walk before?"

"This is my first."

"Ever? You never had a baby die on you before?"

"No. He was my first."

"Well, child, he sure won't be your last. You have a good day now." LaVerne turned to resume her work.

I wiped my eyes as I rode back up to the sixth floor and said a silent prayer for Luke and his parents. As I entered the unit, I saw the end of a bed being wheeled into bed space #9. The charge nurse walked me to the room, filling me in on the details of my new patient, a three-year-old boy with a brain tumor and uncontrolled hypertension. His parents were in the waiting room, anxious and wanting to meet the nurse.

* * * *

A few weeks later a card arrived for me in the pediatric ICU.

> *Dear Colleen,*
>
> *Words cannot express how thankful we are of your care and support to Luke and us during those last three months difficult time, especially your support during the last period of Luke's life had greatly eased our pain.*
>
> *For a nurse to know that her care really helps patients in their difficult time is a great satisfaction to her. That is why I write this note to you, to let you know you are an excellent nurse and to show our gratitude.*
>
> *Love,*
> *Joe & Liu*

Tucked inside the card was a photograph of Luke, taken the day he was born. Eyes open, a full head of jet-black hair, and tiny fists curled up by his cheeks. A perfect, beautiful baby boy.

LaVerne was right, of course. Luke would not be the last child I placed in a parent's grieving arms, but he will remain in my heart as my first. His picture remains safely tucked inside the card from Liu, stored with my most precious possessions.

Oct. 17, 1989

It was a little after 5 pm, and I was on my first cup of coffee. In the middle of a two-week night-shift rotation, I had about ninety minutes before I needed to leave for work. I turned on the TV to watch the pregame show for Game 3 of the World Series, which was being played just a few miles away. San Francisco had eliminated my beloved Cubbies on the way to the Series, and was down to Oakland 2-0.

I listened to Al Michaels as I headed to the kitchen for a refill. I was startled by the rumbling of a large truck rolling by, and as I reached for my coffee pot, I realized the floor was shaking. I looked out towards my living room window and saw my violets fall off the sill. This wasn't a truck going by. I walked towards my television, and Al Michaels was gone, the screen filled first with static, and then with a rerun of *Roseanne*.

I instinctively reached for the phone and called my mom. She answered on the second ring.

"Mom, are you watching TV?"

"Yes- why?"

"Is the World Series on? I was watching it, and the screen went blank. I think we might have had an earthquake."

"Are you okay? Hold on; let me look. No, the game isn't on. Are you okay?"

"I'm fine. I thought it was traffic, but traffic wouldn't keep shaking the building like this." My floor was rolling like I was on a boat.

"Earthquake. You're right. They're saying it was a big one."

"I gotta go, then. It might be hard getting to work." I didn't like the rolling sensation that was still underfoot. It seemed to be lasting too long. Weren't earthquakes short?

"Be careful, okay? Let us know what happens. Love you."

"Love you, too, Mom. I'm fine, and I'll call when I can." As I hung up, the power flickered a few times. I stood against my kitchen counter, trying to decide what to do. After weighing all my options, I decided on a course of action.

I jumped in the shower and washed my hair. It seemed like a good idea, and I wanted to be clean and shampooed if things went south. I did not know how bad the quake had been or what I would be walking into at work, but I knew I would be better equipped for anything that happened if my hair was clean. The power went out while I was in the shower, and I used the last hot water I would have for several days. My blow dryer was not a possibility, so I went to work wearing a leopard print headband.

My fifteen-minute drive took over an hour, and as I reached the top of each hill, I could see smoke coming from the Marina District. Traffic lights were out, traffic was snarled, and it seemed like every few minutes the ground was shaking again. I parked on the street, not wanting to put my car in the garage. It didn't seem safe.

The six flights up to PICU were nothing in comparison to the dozen flights the NICU nurse walking next to me was facing. I arrived on the unit to find that many nurses not scheduled to work had shown up, wanting to help. It was another example of the type of people I was working with. I quickly learned that one of the dayshift nurses no longer had a home. Her basement apartment was now occupied by the top two floors of the building, an old Victorian that had collapsed.

The charge nurse smiled as I approached, "So you're blow dryer dependent, huh?"

"Completely." My hair was limp, and the headband wasn't a good look for me.

"Thanks for coming in. Have a seat, and we'll make you slightly more presentable. Lorrie's mom has offered to help braid the pitiful."

"That would be great." Lorrie was a favorite on the unit. Not yet two years old, she had undergone a bone marrow transplant for leukemia. She had been with us for almost two months, and everyone liked taking care of her. Most children suffered through bone marrow transplants, sickened by the chemo designed to wipe out their immune system so the transplant wouldn't be rejected. Lorrie was a wonderful exception, eating her way through chemotherapy and improving every day. Her mom, Arlene, was popular as well. She spent a great deal of time supporting and encouraging the parents of other children, and she had a contagious positive attitude.

Arlene laughed as she combed my hair. "I didn't know hair could be this flat. No wonder you use a crimper." I had been in a crimping phase for a few months, trying to create volume where none existed. Five minutes later, I was sporting two French braids and a smile. Time to get to work.

THE CHOICE I NEVER HAD TO MAKE

The Loma Prieta earthquake reached a magnitude 7.1. The aftershocks, which came with alarming frequency in the first few days, varied from a definite shaking to a small rolling sensation that made you wonder if it was your imagination. It was hard to tell what was real and what wasn't. I learned to look at the IV bags whenever I felt movement. If it was an aftershock, the IV bags would swing slightly. If they were still, I knew it was in my head.

The hospital had sustained some damage, but as it was explained to us, seismic preparation was part of its design. The buildings actually moved away from each other, and as you climbed to higher floors, the gap between buildings increased. The NICU nurses told us they could see through the gaps in the floor down to the floor below. Our gap was just a few inches on the 6th floor, but as aftershocks continued to occur, structural integrity had to be frequently re-evaluated.

The worst-case scenario was that we would have to evacuate if the building showed signs of failing. I had never really considered the logistics of evacuating from intensive care, but an evacuation plan was in place, and the head nurse spoke with each of us so we would know exactly what to do. I was stunned by what I heard.

"Colleen, your patient is number 16, so if we have to move quickly, you are to go to bed #4 and help Karen."

"I don't understand," I said. "Why would I leave Cody?" Cody was a three year old who had undergone brain surgery to remove a golf-ball-sized tumor. They had been unable to remove it all, and he was facing chemo, radiation, and the possibility of additional surgery. He was having difficulty with increased pressure in his head and was far from stable. I had been taking care of him for several weeks and had bonded with his mother Kasey, a military wife who had absolute faith that she was taking her son home.

"If we have to go quickly, we have to move the children with the best survival chances first. It takes more than one person to move a child, and we have ranked the patients by survivability. If it comes down to it, you will have to leave your child to help save another. I hope to God it doesn't happen, but we have to be ready if it does." She put her hand on my shoulder. "This is worst case, Colleen. If we have to run." She walked away, approaching the nurse beside me, whose child was ranked #3.

Could I leave Cody to help move someone else? I argued both sides of this question in my head. It often took 3-4 people to move one child because of ventilators, pumps, drains, and miscellaneous equipment. A child coming to us from the OR routinely arrived with at least three staff in tow. I understood that it would take multiple people to move each child. Intellectually, it was logical.

But I was a nurse, and this was my patient. How could I leave him behind? My job was to protect him, take care of him, and not do anything to cause harm. Was one life more important the other? No matter how sick a child was, shouldn't it be a level playing field? If it came to an emergency evacuation, would I really be able to walk away from the bedside?

The building remained structurally sound, and no one was evacuated. We stayed put, rolling with the more than 300 aftershocks of magnitude 2.5 or greater that happened in the weeks after the earthquake. We watched our IV bags, looking around to see if anyone else had felt it and hoping they would one day stop happening. Most of all, we gave thanks that we did not have to make a decision about leaving a child behind.

LORRIE

I had three weeks left before my contract ended, and several other travel nurses were getting ready to move on. I was heading to Houston, and my friends were going to Denver, Honolulu, Chicago, and New York. We were scattering, and it was sad to say goodbye. A large group of us, almost the entire night shift, gathered at The Patio Café, one of our favorite places. It catered to hospital employees, offering a $1.99 breakfast and those 99-cent Hot White Russians. Over the course of ten months, we had been there dozens of times.

This was a very special day. Not only were we gathering to say goodbye, we were celebrating the fact that Lorrie was being discharged that morning. She had done amazingly well with her bone marrow transplant and was going home.

"This is what it's all about," I said, "seeing a child go through so much and come out the other side healthy, happy and smiling."

Ann raised her mug, "To Lorrie. The happiest transplant child I have *ever* seen. I've never seen a child eat her way all the way through chemo and a transplant."

"It makes it all worthwhile," Karen said. "This is why we do it. This is why we put those children through the hell of a bone marrow transplant. They do go home."

"And their hair grows back," I added. "Luckily for her, she has a mom who will make the most of each blonde strand that is sprouting."

"To Lorrie! To Arlene, the best hair-braider the peds ICU has ever had!" We had all hugged Arlene on the way out that morning, wishing them both well and thanking her for the love and encouragement she extended to other families. It was a very happy ending.

* * * *

Two weeks later, I watched Cody leave the PICU. He was terminal, and his mother had decided to take him home under the care of hospice. Kasey wanted him to be at home so they could be together as a family for as long as possible. His sister Patty was six years old, and wanted to bake him a birthday cake for his fourth birthday, which was two months away.

I never told Kasey about the night when I learned I might have to leave him behind. She never knew that her son was #16 of sixteen. Her faith was unwavering that she would take him home, and that's exactly what she did. I hoped he would live to see his fourth birthday, and Kasey promised to let me know.

On my very last day in San Francisco, Arlene called the pediatric ICU to let us know that Lorrie had died in her sleep. I was devastated.

HOUSTON, WE HAVE A PROBLEM

I started a thirteen-week contract in the Texas Medical Center, a sprawling complex in the middle of Houston. I was supposed to work in PICU, but the unit was so slow I kept getting sent to neonatal ICU. Unlike Long Island, they did not offer me a rocking chair in the fat farm and routinely gave me assignments for which I felt unqualified. Nursing has many distinct specialties, and being good at one kind of nursing does not make you competent in others.

After several conversations with the nurse recruiter and Keri in Boston, I chose to end my contract and move on. I didn't want to provide mediocre care and certainly did not want to cause harm to a preemie. I wasn't qualified for what they were asking me to do, and I wasn't going to let them pressure me into accepting assignments I wasn't comfortable with. Sometimes, you have to know what you do not know in order to do what's right.

There were no other openings in Houston, so I chose Washington, DC. Keri had told me they had over a dozen travel nurses in the peds ICU, and many of them were extending their contracts. They had just expanded their cardiac surgery program, so my training in San Francisco would be put to good use. Assignments were much more fun if there were lots of other travelers, and I thought that DC would be a great place to be a tourist. It was on my list of expensive cities, and the housing in Alexandria, Virginia was supposed to be really nice.

Memories of San Francisco came rushing back when I got a Christmas card from Kasey. As promised, she let me know what had happened with Cody after taking him home:

Cody had a birthday on November 30th. Patty asked me to bake him a cake to remember him by so I did. I have had you on my mind since getting your last letter, and hope the New Year brings you much happiness, lots of laughter, and most of all, a wonderful, understanding hulk of a man. We love you, Colleen.

Kasey, Robert, Patty and Cody (all the way from heaven)

* * * *

I drove from Houston to DC, stopping to spend a few days with Joan and Henry, Sean's parents. I called them Mom and Dad, and we had been close since I stayed with them after Hurricane Alicia. They had built a house on a lake in Longview, Texas, and I had been told my room would always be ready. As I left their home, Joan told me she wished I was her daughter-in-law. It was something she had told me many times before, but Sean and I never seemed to be on the same page at the same time and had never even dated.

As I continued my drive, I was able to spend an evening with Julie, who was in South Carolina doing a clinical rotation. We had both missed camp that summer and had a fun evening reminiscing. My last stop was at Virginia Tech, where my sister was going to school. We had a nice dinner and filled her mini fridge with snacks, and for the first time in five years, I slept in a dorm. I had to admit I preferred private bathrooms and corporate housing.

I arrived in Alexandria, Virginia in January 1990. My housing was a high rise, and the Pentagon was visible from the balcony. My roommate was in the last week of her assignment, so she gave me a very quick rundown on where to shop, where to bank, the quickest routes across the bridges into DC, and places to avoid. She moved out while I was in hospital orientation, and I had the apartment to myself for two months.

I loved my assignment, which turned out to be a role reversal of sorts. The hospital's pediatric heart program was very new, and the head nurse decided to hire travel nurses with cardiac backgrounds to train the staff. The hospital nurses taught us the hospital policies, and we taught them cardiac care. It worked out very well, and it was fun to go to work.

I hadn't spent as much time as I wanted to in Houston the prior fall, so when my assignment was over, I headed back to Texas. There were no problems this time around. I was in a different and very busy pediatric ICU in the Texas Medical Center, and it was a good assignment. I spent quite a bit of time with Louise, who still lived in Galveston, and was working as the Activities Director for a retirement community.

When the end of my assignment in Houston was nearing, I didn't have a destination in mind. I had been to most of the places I had wanted to see, so was now considering cities based on where I might want to stay when I eventually stopped traveling. I called my recruiter, got a list of available cities, and stared at the map. Where to go? I chose North Carolina, a few hours from my sister and an hour away from the Blue Ridge Parkway, where my parents frequently vacationed.

THE OK CORRAL DIVE CLUB

Things got off to a great start in Winston-Salem. I walked into the pediatric ICU and came face-to-face with Karen, one of the travelers I worked with in San Francisco. She gave me the scoop on the unit, and I had an instant lunch buddy. Karen had four weeks left on her contract, so we did as much as we could in her final weeks. Like me, she was starting to contemplate life after traveling but wanted to finish out the year with one or two more cities. She left for Chicago and met her future husband two weeks later. Karen had found home.

Winston-Salem provided an unusual experience for me because for the first time I made more friends with people who lived there than travelers who were passing through. I became more involved in the community and when I signed up for a scuba course, became close with three of my classmates. We called ourselves the OK Corral Dive Club, a name we came up with on a diving trip to Panama City. The Dive Shop offered discounts to organizations, so we decided to become one right there in their parking lot.

I was especially close with Larry, a DJ for an oldies station who was always up for a road trip or an evening of Jenga. He was fifteen years my senior, and it was a completely platonic friendship. He snuck me into the press box for a Wake Forest football game and got us great seats for music festivals. During a Christmas tree decorating party, fueled by strong eggnog, Larry and his on-air partner recorded my answering machine message:

> *This message is brought to you by Glacier Bay, the official beer of the OK Corral Dive Club. Colleen, also known as a. Dive Goddess, b. Wonder Woman, and c. Queen of Nursing, is not available. If your message is in the least bit interesting, you will hear back from her soon.*

That message stayed on my machine for several years— it was a huge hit among my friends and family and was ultimately retired only because the cassette tape wore out. I really enjoyed my time in North Carolina and went as far as looking at townhomes. I seriously considered purchasing a home and putting down roots. There was a small hitch, however. I really didn't like the hospital, and nursing was not at the level I was now used to. I wrestled with the possibility of roots vs. my love of travel and came up with a win-win solution. I would do both.

COMMUTING

I was five hours away from a hospital I loved, located in a city I would never think of living in permanently. I called the head nurse in Washington, DC and asked if she needed travelers. She said they needed at least three and agreed to let me work seven days on, seven days off. I called my recruiter in Boston, and in September 1990, I became an extreme commuter with two homes.

My housing in DC was paid for, the same high rise with a view of the Pentagon I had lived in before. I established a set routine, spending seven days in DC, working six twelve-hour nights and enjoying one day of rest. I then drove back to North Carolina, where I shared an apartment with a travel nurse who had decided to stay. I had seven days to play in Winston-Salem before returning to work in DC. I had the best of both worlds.

The cardiac program had flourished in DC and was very busy. I almost always worked in the heart room, a large enclosed space with four beds, used exclusively for our open-heart kids. Easter weekend, I was taking care of Chance, a seven-month-old recovering from his second heart surgery. He was struggling, maxed out on every medication that might support his cardiac function. It wasn't enough, and his heart was failing. The cardiologist and heart surgeon were both at the bedside, trying to agree on a course of action.

The heart surgeon was called Dr. Bob by staff and families alike, and when he spoke, people listened. He called down to the OR desk, saying, "Get someone from the pump team up here now. Yes, I know it's three o'clock in the morning, but this kid can't wait. I want a perfusionist, and I want one now."

I knew very little about perfusion. It was a very high tech specialty involving cardiopulmonary support, and perfusionists were not often seen outside of the operating room. I had never worked with one, and thought it would be really interesting to see what could be done at the bedside.

Twenty minutes later, the Chief Perfusionist walked in the door, smoothing his steel gray hair with his fingers and downing an enormous cup of coffee. He was relaxed and confident, and it was clear he had the respect of Dr. Bob. "You rang?"

"Thanks for coming, Steve. Need your input on this one. Chance is in heart failure, but it's not anything I can fix surgically, and he's maxed on drips. I want to give his heart a rest. What can you do here at the bedside?"

Steve walked around the bed, sizing up the space. He was completely unfazed by our middle of the night crisis. "I can modify a pump pack into an ECMO circuit. Would that work for you? Easy enough. I can be ready in fifteen minutes."

Dr. Bob nodded, satisfied with the answer. "Do it. Can you cover this and the OR schedule?"

"It depends." Steve gave me a lazy smile. "Sorry—what's your name?"

"Colleen."

"Well, Colleen. What's the coffee situation up here?"

"Strong, never ending, and brewing as we speak."

"Looks like we are all set, Bob. I'll be back in five, ready in fifteen." He walked towards the door, stopping at the threshold. "Colleen, can you try to get me 4 units of blood in the next fifteen minutes?"

"I have two here, and I'll work on two more."

He nodded. "And a beautiful friendship was born."

Fifteen minutes later, Chance was being supported by the ECMO circuit. ECMO, extracorporeal membrane oxygenation, was a treatment that used a pump to circulate blood through an artificial lung. It supported the heart and lungs, giving them time to heal. Many hospitals had ECMO teams staffed by nurses, but this hospital didn't. Steve chose to work the overnight shift in PICU, allowing his staff to keep the OR running smoothly. We were within ten feet of each other for 3 ½ shifts, and I learned about perfusion.

The primary role of a perfusionist was to run the heart-lung machine during open-heart surgery. Bypass took place in the OR, while ECMO took place in ICU. Steve could explain it in one sentence. "The purpose of ECMO is to allow time for the heart and lungs to recover, and standard cardiopulmonary bypass provides support during various types of cardiac surgical procedures." I heard him explain this over and over as nurses came to see the modified circuit Steve had built. I asked about his training and how a person might become a perfusionist.

"You need to start applying two years before you plan on going," he said. "Programs are very competitive, and it is hard to get in. Most people apply everywhere and go wherever they are accepted." *Everywhere* turned out to be only fifteen programs in the entire country.

It gave me something to think about, and I kept it in the back of my mind as I contemplated my next move. I had been splitting my time between two cities for almost nine months, and while I liked working in DC and playing in Winston-Salem, it was time to live and work in the same place.

I found myself once again staring at the map, considering my options. I had been to the expensive cities I had wanted to live in and had spent enough time in different parts of the country to know where I *didn't* want to go. Almost certain that I would be retiring from travel nursing in the near future, I chose to go where many retirees went: Florida.

RETIREMENT

My last assignment was in St. Petersburg, Florida. My paternal grandparents lived there, and the drive across one of the Tampa Bay bridges brought back happy memories of visiting as a child. My brothers and sister and I would get really excited when we crossed the bridge because it meant we were almost there. The pelicans and seagulls still made me smile, and I was glad to be back, wanting to spend more time with my grandparents.

The hospital I worked at had two pediatric ICUs, one medical and one surgical. I was placed in the medical PICU, working twelve-hour nights. I was the only travel nurse and didn't meet many nurses who were looking for a new friend. It was cordial but not welcoming. The hospital was excellent, but I missed working with open heart kids and knew very quickly that I would not want to become a staff nurse. What to do?

In talking with many of the travelers I worked with, it seemed we shared a common problem. How do you stop traveling? How do you settle into one place, doing things one way, when you know there are a dozen different ways of accomplishing the same task? As a travel nurse, I got to decide when and where I worked. That freedom was not to be found as a staff nurse. I realized that I would not be happy without a new challenge, so I decided to do what several of my travel friends were doing: go back to school.

While my friends were choosing to become nurse practitioners or nurse anesthetists, I chose perfusion. Steve had shown me a whole new world, and I wanted to try my hand as a CCP, a Certified Clinical Perfusionist. Steve had been right about the difficulty in getting into perfusion school. It took eighteen months to get into the school I wanted to attend, and I worked as a home health nurse while waiting to get started.

In January 1992, I bundled up and moved to Pittsburgh, Pennsylvania.

BACK TO SCHOOL

At the ripe old age of twenty-nine, I learned how to study. Our first subject was cardiac physiology, a subject in which I thought I was well-versed. The reading assignment totaled 625 pages, and I realized nothing I had done before arriving in Pittsburgh had prepared me for the challenge of perfusion school. Days were long, starting before sunrise and stretching well into the evenings. We were responsible for all readings and coursework on our own time after completing a full day in the operating room. I worked hard to learn the mountains of material we were given, as did my classmates.

Only four of us had been accepted into school, and we quickly bonded. Scott and Marc were both married, and their wives joined in whenever we got together. Christine was an adult ICU nurse, and we became very close over double cappuccinos at the coffee house halfway between our apartments. We puzzled over Pittsburghese, the local slang we were learning that included "yunz." It was similar to "Y'all" and "you guys" but never sounded natural coming out of our mouths.

There was no time to visit the sights of Pittsburgh, and I rarely left the neighborhood I lived in. I was six blocks from the hospital, and as I trudged through snow that reached well above my boots during one of many blizzards that winter, I questioned my decision-making process.

Against the advice of my program director, I took a part-time job as a home health nurse, working every Saturday. I read fluid dynamics to the ten-month-old child I took care of, and as long as I did it in a sing-song voice, she didn't seem to mind. I found work to be relaxing and added monthly visits at a nursing home down the street from my apartment. On the last Sunday of the month, I visited three ladies who each needed an injection. That one hour of work, which included quite a bit of chit-chat, supported my coffee habit.

Christine, Marc, Scott, and I all started looking for jobs six months before we graduated. The job market was tight, and we were advised to take whatever job we were offered, knowing that it would probably be a temporary situation. Perfusion was a young specialty, and many of the original perfusionists were still working. The reality was that the best jobs were taken by long-term employees, and you had to wait until they retired before a position became available. The turnover took place in hospitals where the work conditions were less than ideal. Each of us had a specific part of the country in mind, which made job-hunting even more challenging.

Overall, we did pretty well. Scott, who was from Memphis, ended up in Tupelo, Mississippi. Marc was aiming for Wyoming and landed a position in Colorado. Christine found a job in the Philadelphia suburbs, and much to my surprise, I was headed back to Florida. I'd contacted the chief cardiac surgeon in St. Petersburg, and even though there were no openings, he agreed to meet with me. I took a quick trip to Florida, and when we met, he asked why I wanted to move back to St. Petersburg. I told him about my grandparents and my long-time affection for the area, and it turned out that he used to be a customer at my grandfather's fishing tackle store. He offered me a job on the spot. It was a part-time position with the possibility of becoming full time, and I gratefully accepted the offer.

Scott's wife was a caterer and made beautifully decorated cakes. Each of us had been treated to the cake of our choice on our birthday, and as we got together for our last goodbyes, she presented us with a cake we had joked about while celebrating our last exam. It was Mount Rushmore, with our faces replacing those of the presidents. Parked below the monument were our four cars, packed with luggage and sporting a banner across the bumper. Mine said "Florida or bust." See yunz later.

PERFUSION

I worked in St. Petersburg for a year and a half. I spent a great deal of time with my grandparents and passed both my written and oral board exams, earning my CCP certification. When it became apparent that the heart program would not be expanding enough to support a full-time position, I moved on, accepting a full time job in Jacksonville.

Jacksonville was one of the worst mistakes of my professional life. I had visited as part of the interview process and had dinner with one of the two surgeons and all of the perfusionists. We toured the OR after hours, which I should have recognized as a huge red flag. The first time I stepped into the operating room as a new employee I was stunned by the behaviors I saw. It epitomized a hostile work environment, with nurses being screamed at, obscenities flowing like water, and a total lack of professionalism. I started looking for perfusion job #3 as soon as I got home. My contract included a ninety-day probationary period that allowed both parties to terminate without notice, and on day forty, I gave my two weeks' notice.

Next stop, Louisville, KY. Jacksonville wasn't a total loss by any stretch of the imagination. I met my future husband during the move to Louisville, so if I hadn't gone to Jacksonville, I wouldn't have met Thomas. He walked up to my front door and knocked, smiling at me when I opened the door, asking "Are you ready for me?"

Sign me up, I thought, but answered with a simple "Sure, come on in."

He was one of my movers, and over the course of a few hours, we talked as much as was possible with him carrying my furniture down the stairs. I found him to be funny, personable, and very confident. As he said goodbye, he asked if he could buy me dinner in Louisville after my things had been unloaded. I said if everything arrived unbroken, I would cook for him. We shook on it, and he hugged me.

He was my silver lining, and I arrived in Louisville with high hopes. I was working with a large perfusion group, and a new pediatric heart surgeon had just been brought in to expand the children's heart program. I was one of three perfusionists who did kids and had been hired specifically because of the expansion.

Thomas didn't leave Louisville after unloading my furniture and taking me to dinner. On Christmas Eve, seventy-two days after we met, we were married in my parents' living room, standing next to the Christmas tree. Things were looking great. I was working in a good hospital, had a husband I was very much in love with, and was only five hours away from my family in Chicago. Time to put down some roots.

INTRODUCTION TO DEMENTIA

I was taking my world-famous, poppy-seed chicken out of the oven when the phone rang. It was my grandfather, calling from St. Pete, and his voice sounded strained. The fact that he was calling was highly unusual because my grandfather rarely spoke on the phone. Whenever I called, he handed the phone to my grandmother within the first minute or so, saying "Talk to your grandma."

"What's wrong, Grandpa? You sound worried."

"It's Ella. I don't know what to do." I had never heard my grandfather say that— he *always* knew what to do.

"Tell me what's going on, and I'll try to help."

His voice shook. "She doesn't know who I am. I walked out of the kitchen, and she asked me who I was. I think she's afraid of me."

"Where is she?" I was trying to think of a way I could help from 900 miles away.

"She's in the bedroom, sitting at the foot of the bed. Every time I try to go in, she asks who I am and goes into her closet. I don't know what to do. What should I do?" The fear in his voice was heartbreaking.

"Do you think she will pick up the phone? Maybe I can talk to her and get an idea of what is going on." It was worth a try, I thought.

She wouldn't take the phone from Grandpa, so I asked him to hang up, put the bedroom phone on their bed, walk out into the living room and sit on the couch. I would call and see if she answered.

It worked. Grandma answered on the 3rd ring. "Hello?"

"Hi, Grandma, it's Colleen. How are you?"

"Just fine, darling, good to hear your voice. Are you coming over on Sunday?" She didn't seem to know I had moved six months ago.

"Sorry, but no. I have to work this weekend. Is there a man walking around your condo, Grandma?"

"He's been here all day, but I don't know who he is. He says he's my husband, but he doesn't look a thing like him."

"Can you do me a favor, Grandma?"

"Of course. Anything."

I could only think of one thing to do. "Could you go out into the living room and pick up that big picture sitting on top of the TV? It's the picture taken for the church directory."

"Okay. Do you want me to send it to you?"

"No. I want you to look at the man in that photograph. Does he look familiar?"

"It's your Grandpa. Why?"

I hoped this would work. "Take a good look at the man sitting on the couch and then look at that picture. Does it look like the same man, Grandma?"

"I guess so."

"Grandma, I promise you that the man sitting on your couch is your husband and my grandfather. You don't have to worry or be nervous. It's just Grandpa."

There was a brief pause, and I waited, hoping.

"Well, dear. I guess I'll have to take your word for it. He doesn't look a thing like my husband, though."

"I love you, Grandma, and promise that man is your husband. Everything is just fine."

"Okay, dear. Nice to hear your voice."

"Can I talk to the man on the couch? Grandpa?" I could only imagine what he must be feeling.

"Okay. Will I see you on Sunday?"

"I'll try, Grandma. Love you."

"Love you, too."

I told my grandfather what I had said and suggested he make an appointment with their doctor. He asked if he could call again if he needed me, and I told him he could call anytime, day or night.

He called me three nights in a row, and I had the same conversation with my grandmother. Each time she said, "Well, I guess I'll take your word for it, dear" when I told her the man in her house was her husband.

On the fourth night, my grandmother answered on the 3rd ring, and when I said, "Hi Grandma, it's Colleen," she said, "Do I know you?"

And that is how dementia entered my life.

SEPTEMBER 11, 2001

My husband Thomas was a New Yorker born in the Bronx and was thrilled when I was offered a position in Manhattan. Just as I had been warned back in Pittsburgh, it could take several attempts to find a permanent home as a perfusionist. Louisville's pediatric program had been a failure, and I was downsized out of my next job in Virginia when a competing hospital bought out the heart program. I had been offered a job on the pediatric heart team at a large teaching hospital in NYC and decided to try again. This was my fifth perfusion job in eight years, and I was wondering if I would ever find a home.

I was lucky that Thomas shared my sense of adventure. He was supportive of each move and told me he could be happy anywhere as long as we were together. As a jack-of-all-trades, he never had a problem finding a job, and when New York became a possibility, he was really excited. He loved the New York Giants and Yankees as much as I loved the Chicago Bears and Cubs and told me he would protect me when I wore my Chicago gear into New York stadiums. If I wasn't on-call, we went to Yankees games, and they were really fun. The ladies rooms were pink in Yankee stadium, which I thought was a nice touch.

We lived on the Upper East Side. I had to be within twenty minutes of the hospital when on call and in New York that could be just a few blocks away. We were in hospital housing, using every square inch of our 440 square feet. We joked about it being a test of how much we really liked each other and discovered the joys of IKEA as we downsized from a three-bedroom house into the tiny apartment.

Thomas was working as an ironworker, specialized in fencing. He fenced baseball stadiums, bridges, parking lots, and rooftops. He had just finished a project and was waiting for his next job. On the morning of September 11th, he headed to the Union Hall on West

42nd Street. I drove out to Queens, NY because I was covering maternity leave for a perfusionist in our sister hospital. I was in the OR by 6:30 am. We had two heart surgeries on the schedule.

I was on bypass at 8:46 am when a plane hit the North Tower of the World Trade Center. No one in our operating room suite had any idea of what was happening. At 9:03 am, when the South Tower was hit, we were hearing conflicting stories about bombs, planes, and air traffic control failures.

Someone stuck their head in the door, announcing "The Pentagon is burning."

The surgeon yelled, "Get out! Focus people! We have a job to do."

We did our jobs, finished the surgery, and readied to transfer our patient to the ICU. The next patient was having some blood sugar issues, so the 2nd heart surgery of the day was on hold until the surgeon and anesthesiologist could assess the patient in the holding area. As we rolled out of the OR, we were met with a wave of confusion and panic.

The realization that our lives had been changed came in snippets of information. Nurses marry firemen and cops, and many of the OR staff had family that would be first responders. Cell phones were brought out, and "Do you have a signal? Are there any bars?" was repeated throughout the halls. The hospital phone system was working but people were told not to use it.

I walked back towards the OR, and my phone beeped, indicating I had a message. It was Thomas. "Hey Coll, there's been explosions at the towers. Everyone is leaving the Hall and heading downtown. We have guys on the roof, and we're going to get them. Love you."

I tried to call him, but it didn't go through. Trying to focus on work, I headed towards the holding room to find out what was happening with the next surgery. A nurse stopped me in the hall. "Did you hear?"

"About the case? Has it been cancelled?" With everything going on, it was odd that I assumed she was talking about the second surgery.

"No. The South Tower is gone."

"What do you mean it's gone?" I didn't understand.

"It collapsed, and it's totally gone." She was pale, and I remembered that her brother was a firefighter.

"Were people still inside? Had it been evacuated?" How could the entire South Tower disappear? I had been on the rooftop observation deck several times and couldn't comprehend a building of that size collapsing into lower Manhattan.

Then it hit me. Thomas. Which tower was he rushing into? Was he there? Was he hurt? Was he alive? I was one of many people standing in shock, wondering if they had lost a loved one. And none of us had answers. I remember thinking that *surely* I would know if he was dead.

When I got to the holding room, people were gathered round the TV, which was showing images of a smoking tower. The director of the OR walked into the room and turned the TV off. "Listen up, people. Time to get ready for casualties. Let's get to work. We will pass along information as we get it."

I was able to call my boss in Manhattan using the hospital phone system. He told me that the bridges and tunnels had been closed and that he needed me to stay there for the duration. "We don't know how many people we will get, Colleen, so make sure you are ready for traumas, have extra circuits ready, and do the best you can. We'll get someone out there when we can, but for now, you need to work with what you have." I had one other perfusionist in the building, and she needed to be supervised.

"Okay. I'll stay close to the office in case you have news. Right now, we are on hold with scheduled surgeries." I made a request before hanging up. "Thomas was heading to the towers with other ironworkers, and I don't know where he is. If anyone hears from him, let me know, okay?" Thomas had the number to the perfusion office in Manhattan, and I hoped he would think to call there if he couldn't reach my cell.

"Will do. Good luck." He hung up, and I very quickly called my parents, telling them I was okay but did not know where Thomas was or if he had been in the tower when it collapsed. I asked them to pray and told them I loved them. That was the last time I was able to reach them for several days.

The North Tower collapsed, and people started hearing about confirmed deaths. You could hear cries echoing down the hall as wives lost husbands, mothers lost children, and sisters lost brothers. The most repeated words that day were "Have you heard? Do you know?"

Was it better to know or not know? We were marking time, waiting for trauma patients. The OR director told us we would be housed in the 6th floor pedi unit. It was vacant and scheduled for renovations, so we could use the rooms while we stayed on trauma call. As we understood it, the city-wide plan was that hospitals would be filled by proximity to the scene, and as hospitals filled, they would expand out towards the boroughs. We would not see patients until the expansion reached Queens.

I stayed in the OR until dinnertime, sitting with my coworkers, waiting for news. After checking my supplies one last time, I collected soap, a toothbrush, and toothpaste from the ICU. They had opened their patient supply closet so people could take what they needed. I walked upstairs to the vacant unit I would call home for the next few days.

I don't know where they came from, but twin sized air mattresses were lining the halls, and two linen carts provided sheets and towels. I dragged a mattress into one of the rooms, which was empty except for a metal crib, the kind I had worked with as a pediatric nurse. I lowered the rails and piled my linens on the hospital-issue thin green mattress. Walking to the west facing window, I could see the plumes of smoke rising over lower Manhattan.

As it grew dark, there was a surreal glow hovering over where the towers should be. There were scattered power outages in the city, and the famous skyline looked broken. I stared into the night, wondering where Thomas was, and reassuring myself that if he was gone my heart would know.

It was one the longest nights of my life. I did not sleep, and I let my mind wander as I lay on an air mattress, wedged against the crib. I said prayers for Thomas and for all of us who were waiting. I thought about my parents, who I knew would be praying. I replayed happy memories and gave thanks for what I had. I got up several times to look out the window, hoping each time I would see something different.

I thought about Burt in LA, wondering if he found happiness after suffering such severe burns at the hands of his father. I thought about Luke, remembering the elevator ride to the morgue. And Lorrie, who we thought had beaten the odds. I remembered the looks on the faces of my campers as I defeated the alligator, and the laughter I had shared with other travelers as we tried to cram as much fun into thirteen weeks as we possibly could. I thought about Jake, David, Charlie, and Voodoo Mary, wondering if any of them had achieved a normal life.

As dawn broke, I had an epiphany. In spending a night thinking about everything that mattered to me, it came down to nursing. I had not thought about perfusion at all. Not once. My heart was where it always had been, and I simply hadn't noticed. I was a nurse and needed to get back to nursing.

September 12th passed in heart-wrenching slow motion. Information was limited and communication was erratic. More and more of my coworkers learned that they had lost a loved one, and good news did not seem to be coming. At 9:00 pm, the phone in the perfusion office rang. It was Stan, a perfusionist who had started the same week I had. We were friends, and his fiancé was a travel nurse. We had double dated on several occasions, and he and Thomas often went to the gym together.

"Colleen, I have someone who wants to say hello."

"Thomas? Is that you? Are you okay?"

"Coll? Can you hear me? I'm okay! I'm okay!" It was very difficult to hear, but it was Thomas. "We are trying to dig people out. I borrowed someone's phone and called Stan when your phone went straight to voicemail. It's unbelievable. You can't imagine --."

"Thomas?"

Stan answered. "He was on my cell, and we lost the connection. I had my cell pressed against the office phone so you could hear his voice. He's okay, Colleen."

"Thank you so much, Stan. I was beginning to doubt my gut. It's been thirty-six hours, and most people are getting bad news."

"You holding the fort?"

"We're just waiting," I said. "Have you gotten survivors?"

"No. I don't think we will be getting any. I have to go; I'm not supposed to be using this line. Be safe, ok?"

"You, too."

Stan was right. We did not get a single casualty, and on the morning of September 13th, one of the heart surgeons drove me back to Manhattan. Physicians were allowed to cross the bridges. Thomas was waiting for me in front of our apartment. We hugged for a very long time, and he returned to Ground Zero, where he volunteered until the cleanup was organized.

We were both profoundly changed by the events of September 11th. Three months later I was back in nursing, working with developmentally disabled adults and children.

WORK WITH WHAT YOU ARE GIVEN

Sharon was quite possibly the best nurse I ever worked with. As Director of Nursing for a large agency serving thousands of adults and children with developmental disabilities, she was responsible for overseeing nursing services in all day programs and residential settings. When I interviewed with her, I had the feeling we would be a very good team.

We were opposites with a common center. I had the obsessive organization of a peds ICU nurse and was good at translating ideas into policies. I liked to teach, write, and focus on the details. Sharon was in a state of constant clutter. She carried two oversized bags everywhere she went, and they overflowed with random documents, samples of supplies, reference material, and lots of hair accessories. Within her "bag lady chaos" as she called it, she knew exactly what needed to be done. We shared fierce protectiveness of every person under our care, a desire to always make things better, and a genuine love for this population of people. In New York, the politically correct term for participants in developmental disability programs was "consumer."

I eventually became the nurse educator, training all new employees on health policies, first aid, adapting to the unique needs of our people, and the importance of allowing each individual to flourish. I served on the human rights committee and helped with investigations. It was a wonderful job, and I felt like I was making a difference. In developmental disabilities, I found everything I had been missing in my time as a perfusionist.

I watched as Sharon encouraged staff members to go back to school, to improve their skills, and to find their unique strengths. She could find something positive in an employee that was struggling, and by encouraging that aspect, she improved their job performance and their attitude.

I asked her about this skill I admired, and she told me it was very simple. "We are asking people to do hard work for low wages, long hours, and less thanks than they deserve. There is not an endless supply of people willing to do this job, so it is up to us to help each person be the best they can possibly be. If you work with what you are given, develop the talents that each person possesses, and let them know they are valued, everyone wins."

In working with Sharon, I became a much better nurse. I laughed every day and loved the population I was working with. I tried to apply her philosophy to all aspects of my life. Don't we all want to feel as if others recognize our value?

SEIZING BY THE BAY

Spring Formal was one of the most anticipated nights of the year. It was an agency-wide formal dinner dance held at Russo's on the Bay, a beautiful waterfront restaurant and banquet hall in Queens. Our consumers looked forward to it for months, and the hair and makeup sessions the day of the party were some of my favorite moments of the year.

There were several hundred people in attendance, a nice mix of staff, consumers, family members, and supporters of the agency. We had a delicious dinner, and then the entertainment began. The dance floor filled, and Thomas was pulled onto the floor by a sixty-two year old woman who attended one of the day programs I worked with. Thomas had visited me at work many times and was a hit with the ladies.

My dance card stayed full, and my partners varied from young men in wheelchairs, older guys with interesting moves, a few male staff members, and some of the ladies.

I was dancing with Ed, a twenty-eight year old consumer from the day habilitation program. He had a mild developmental disability that came with some aggressive behaviors and had a habit of using his two hundred-fifty plus pounds and 6'3" frame to intimidate people. He tried that with me when I was new to the agency, and when I climbed onto a chair in order to look him in the eyes, he had laughed, saying, "Nurse Colleen, you are crazy. Let me help you off that chair."

Respect was earned with Ed. That seemed to do the trick, and we developed a good relationship. As we danced to a Michael Jackson song, he gave me what to him was a huge compliment. "Nurse Colleen, you dance really good for a white girl."

"Thanks, Ed. Trying to represent."

"Nurse Colleen, you're crazy. Wait a minute." He stopped dancing in the middle of the song and pointed across the room.

"They need you, Nurse Colleen."

I stopped dancing and looked toward the back of the room. A few staff members were standing in a circle, waving me over. I wound my way through the crowd and arrived to find one of our consumers on the floor having a seizure. In spite of multiple medications, Ellen had seizures pretty regularly. Hers involved dropping to the ground and having small jerking movements in her arms and legs. I sat beside her and told her everything was okay.

I didn't need to intervene because she was safe, and her seizures were consistently time limited. I was just there to make sure it wasn't a new kind of seizure or one that went unusually long and became an emergent situation. Some of our guests that evening didn't understand that seizures were sometimes commonplace, and 911 had been called.

EMS personnel kneeled down and started with a barrage of questions, directing people to stand back. Ellen's best friend Vivian wasn't going anywhere. She tapped one of the EMS guys on the shoulder, not letting up until she had his attention. He looked up at her, taking in her mint green ball gown and the glittery tiara, which was now slightly askew on her head. Vivian had Down's syndrome and stood at slightly over five-feet tall. She and Ellen had been best friends for decades and lived in the same group home.

"You need to back-off, mister. Ellen has seizures. No big deal. She has them, they end, and life goes on. She doesn't need an ambulance because nothing is wrong with her. She's gonna want to dance, so just back off."

The EMS guy looked at me, raising an eyebrow. I could see the smile he was trying to conceal. His partner failed in his attempts to remain professional and was laughing loudly, reaching over to give Vivian a high five.

My response was brief and to the point. "What she said."

EMS left after a few forms were signed, and our evening continued. Ellen sat in a chair at the edge of the dance floor, and Vivian danced with her until the music ended.

I was fortunate to attend Spring Formals for three years in a row and loved my job. Life had other plans for me, however, and I was faced with a difficult choice. Thomas had become a different person since September 11th, increasingly angry and rarely relaxed. He started fighting with neighbors over parking spaces and drinking heavily with his friends. My marriage was crumbling, and I knew if we stayed in New York things would only get worse. In a last ditch effort to right the ship, we left New York for a simpler, quieter life in Florida.

LEGAL NURSING

When we moved to St. Petersburg, I decided to pursue a completely different path into a career I had been encouraged to pursue by an attorney I met about six weeks before we moved.

As part of my job as a nurse educator in New York, I presented an argument for obtaining consent for cataract surgery for a sixty-two year old man who was profoundly developmentally disabled. Since he could not give informed consent, the agency had to obtain the approval from a committee designed to protect his rights. It was my job to present the reasons for doing the surgery, the risks versus benefits, and a detailed account of how cataracts were affecting his quality of life.

After I had successfully lobbied for consent, I was approached by a lawyer who sat on the committee. "I didn't know your agency had legal nurses."

"We don't," I said.

"Actually, I think you are one," he responded, "and I would love to have you look at a case I am evaluating." I agreed to look at it, saw the problems right away, and wrote a summary for him. Just like that, I began my career as a legal nurse consultant.

I went to Las Vegas to take a week-long course on legal nursing. There were over two hundred nurses taking the course, and it was an enthusiastic group. I paid attention, took notes, and studied each evening. I was fortunate to sit next to Maura, a nurse from Reno who I liked right away. We went out to dinner a few times and talked about our dreams of having flexibility and freedom in our schedules while making a good living doing something we both liked and were good at. For me, that was the whole point. I loved the idea of working for myself and thought that if I could build a successful business, it would give me time to do other things I cared about.

During one of my dinners with Maura, we talked about ways of getting our businesses up and running and how we would market our work. How could we best describe what we could offer? I had a thought. "In essence, we will convince attorneys to pay us to critique other people's job performance and actions. I've done that for free since becoming a nurse!"

After she stopped laughing, Maura added, "I don't think that's the slogan you should put on your business card, but it's a good point. We just have to get attorneys to recognize what we offer."

I knew that I would be good at legal nursing because it fed into every obsessively-compulsively-organized trait I possessed. It was a career in which I could both focus on the details and present the big picture in a clear, cohesive manner. I left Las Vegas feeling as if I could rule the world (or at least a part of St. Petersburg, Florida).

The lack of a paycheck is great motivation towards building a successful business, and three months after arriving in Florida, I had developed a respectable workload. I tried many different types of marketing and found that mailings, cold calls, and the "direct" approach did not work nearly as well for me as networking did.

I joined several networking groups in which people from all types of fields got together once a week to provide information about their businesses and learn about the businesses of the other members. We helped each other succeed by providing referrals whenever possible. I found these groups very helpful with honing-in on the way I described my work. We were each given thirty seconds to stand up and give our "elevator speech," which is, in essence, a compact, interesting description of the service you provide.

I found a description that worked well. "How many of you have ever been to a doctor's office or hospital and had a physician give an explanation of what is going on?"

Every person raised a hand, and I continued. "Once the doctor leaves the room, what usually happens?" I paused for a minute before answering my own question. "They all look at the nurse and ask, 'What did he say?'"

People smiled. "That's what I do for attorneys. I evaluate medical records and describe who did what to whom in plain

English." The nodding heads in the room told me I had found an elevator speech that would work for me.

I worked from home, went to lots of networking events, and found myself specializing in personal injury. When I started my business, I thought I would work mainly on medical malpractice cases, but I seemed to connect more easily with personal injury and wrongful death attorneys. Business was steady, and I continued to reach out to additional attorneys, knowing that expanding my client base was important.

On a particularly hot and humid September day, I was struggling through an awkward meeting with Mike, a potential client. We weren't communicating well, and I found myself wishing he would turn down the thermostat because his office was oppressively warm. When he asked me for the third time to explain exactly what I could put in a report, I gave him an answer very different than the ones I had already tried.

"I can give you the good, the bad, and the ugly so you can base decisions on the whole story."

I saw it register in his eyes. He got it. We were finally communicating, and I left his office with a case. When I delivered my report three days later, he was pleased with it and gave me three more files.

A few days later my phone rang, and an unfamiliar voice spoke rapidly into my ear. "This is Matthew, and I need one of those GBUs of yours."

I was clueless. "I'm sorry, what? I'm not following you. Have we met?"

"No. Mike is a friend of mine. He brought your GBU thingy to lunch the other day, and I need a few of those done. How do we make that happen?"

"A GBU?" I still wasn't sure what we were talking about.

"Yeah, a GBU. The good, the bad, and the ugly."

"We can make that happen very easily, Matthew," I responded. "How's your schedule tomorrow?"

Over the course of the next week, I heard from every attorney that had been at the lunch table with Mike. When they asked for a GBU, I knew exactly what they wanted, and these reports quickly became my bread and butter. My business blossomed with the good, the bad, and the ugly, one GBU thingy at a time.

WASHINGTON STATE

A change in geography did nothing to help my marriage, and after twelve years together, Thomas and I divorced. In many ways, my marriage was a casualty of 9/11. I'm sure I am not alone in experiencing that result. There are many, many living victims of that day, and most of us cannot begin to understand the extent of the damage that was done. Thomas wasn't willing to get help in dealing with the trauma he suffered when volunteering at Ground Zero, and I had to accept that I could not save him. It was a heartbreaking decision, but I knew I had gone as far as I could down the path he was taking and had to save myself.

I started my new life as a divorced forty-something by reaching back into my past, hoping to catch up with friends lost along the way. Sean and I reconnected once again and unexpectedly found ourselves dating. He was in Seattle, and I was in Florida, and after a year of cross-country visits, I took a leap of faith. I moved to Washington, hoping for a fresh start and the possibility of happily-ever-after.

I loved Washington and was fortunate to work with a few local attorneys. My out-of-state clients kept sending me work, so business was steady. On a beautiful May afternoon, Sean and I took a drive to the coast, stopping for dinner at one of our favorite restaurants. At the table next to us, there was a family of four, and one of the kids was in a wheelchair. I smiled at her as I passed, and the smile she gave me in return reminded me immediately of one of my campers from Illinois. I told Sean about my summers at camp and how much I had loved it.

The next morning, I perused the help wanted ads in the Sunday paper while enjoying my second cup of coffee. A small ad caught my eye. I had *déjà vu* as four lines jumped off the page:

Camp for special needs children and adults is looking for a registered nurse. Five-week commitment needed, and experience with developmentally and/or physically disabled populations preferred. If interested, please call.

I couldn't stop smiling, and four days later accepted the job.

COFFEE, CONVERSATIONS &
GLOVES IN JULY

I wrapped my fingers around the welcome warmth of the coffee mug. It was one of those chilly July mornings in Washington State. Chilly July mornings—a surprise that had left me unprepared and scrambling for gloves during the last session. I was well-stocked now, though, and had handed them out to my campers the night before when temperatures dipped into the 50s.

It was a little after 7 am. The sun was slow in warming the morning, and I headed to the breakfast tent for a refill. I was in the habit of being ready with morning medications well before most of the staff and campers were awake, and only a few people were up and dressed. Like me, they had gravitated towards coffee, and as I doctored my cup, I listened to the conversation at the table closest to the coffeepot.

"How are things at home?"

Chris, absorbed in trying to pull a wisp of yarn from the glove tip of his left index finger, didn't look up as he answered. "Not bad. Same-old, same-old. People coming and going, trying to follow the rules, keep the peace, share the remote. You know how it is."

Bobby nodded. "I hear ya. How's the food?"

"Depends. Some people cook better than others. You can tell every morning if it is a good food day or not. It all depends, my man."

The string would not come loose, so Chris tried biting it off, continuing to speak as he chewed on his fingertip. "There's this girl who cooks on the weekend. Most of her food you just want to throw away. Or hide. Sometimes, I put it in my pocket. If I had a dog, I would feed it to my dog. I just don't know if he would eat it. Guess you should be nice to your dog, though, and bad food really isn't nice."

Triumph. Chris held the offending length of red yarn between his thumb and index finger, showing it proudly to his friend. He glanced my way, took a sip of coffee, and smiled as he gave me a thumbs up. I returned the gesture, raising a thumb clad in hot pink, agreeing that coffee was a wonderful thing.

Returning his attention to his friend, Chris asked, "How are things with your mom these days?"

Bobby sighed, resting his head in his hands. "It's tough, buddy. She tells me what to do, goes in my room, thinks I should eat brussel sprouts. Carrots I can live with, but brussel sprouts? I don't like 'em. What's a guy to do, though? She's my mom." The fingers of his neon green gloves poked through his hair as he sadly shook his head back and forth. He sighed again.

Chris shook his head, commiserating. "Sorry to hear that, my friend. That's rough."

"Thanks. Sorry your food's bad on the weekend."

"What can you do? That's the way it is, man. Right, Nurse Colleen? That's just the way it is."

I joined them, taking a seat at the table. I loved these early morning chats with my campers. Chris, 61, had cerebral palsy and lived in a group home. Bobby, 52, had Down's syndrome and lived with his mother. We raised our cups in a silent show of unity. Coffee, conversation, and stylish gloves in July. That's the way it should be.

FIELD TRIP

Thursday was the day we went to the community pool— an undertaking that required a school bus, two vans, and several cars. It typically took us about forty-five minutes to get everyone loaded, take attendance, and hit the road for a beautiful twenty minute drive through the Olympic Peninsula.

I was always the last one to leave, bringing up the rear, my car packed with first aid kits, medication, medical information on every camper and counselor, and, of course, my walkie-talkie. It went everywhere with me and allowed me to stay in touch with all of the "red shirts," the term used for the staff with supervisory roles. The fact that we always wore red shirts made us pretty easy to spot.

It was fun to caravan to the pool, and upon arriving we swiftly unloaded, coordinating the staff so every camper was in view while we started the process of getting into the pool one person at a time. Wheelchairs, poor coordination, excitement, and anxiety all came into play. It could take several staff members to get one person into the pool with a bottleneck of excited campers building as they waited to climb in as soon as the steps were clear.

My role at the pool was to brief the lifeguards about any campers I thought might need extra attention, help with loading/unloading campers into the mechanical lift that lowered them into the water, and circle the pool while campers were swimming. I did a continuous head count and watched for signs of fatigue, agitation, dropping body temps, and counselors who might need an extra hand. I watched everything and everyone, and it was a wonderful show.

When everyone who wanted to swim was in the pool, my head count was thirty-one. As usual, there were a few that chose to sit on the side of the pool or in a chair safely away from the splashing. Ruby, 30 years old and a veteran camper, had opted not to get in because it was her time of the month. Never shy, she decided to share this information with James, the twenty-two year old program director.

"James!" She yelled across the pool, her voice echoing off the walls.

Not aware of what was coming, James looked over and gave her a thumbs up.

"James! James! I'm not getting in the pool because *I'm on the rag!*"

Her words bounced, echoed, and seemed to settle over the pool, causing more than a few male counselors to freeze with stunned expressions on their faces. I saw Robert, one of the counselors, go underwater. He was a lifeguard as well and had learned one of the tricks of the trade, submerging when you want to laugh without being seen. I loved watching the counselors when campers said things that were unexpected, or, better yet, totally inappropriate.

Just in case anyone had missed her announcement, Ruby repeated herself at an even higher decibel level. "Did you hear me, James? I'm not getting in the pool *'cause I'm on the rag!*"

To his credit, James kept a straight face and responded with an "Okay, thank you for sharing." I watched him take a few steps behind the bleachers before doubling over.

I kept Ruby company as I watched the pool, using a watering can to sprinkle her legs so she got a little of the pool experience. She had parked her wheelchair about two feet from the edge of the pool, and both staff and campers visited from the water. Within twenty minutes, I saw some of our thinner campers starting to shiver, and the process was reversed, with one camper at a time being helped out of the pool and taken into the changing rooms.

We took advantage of the showers, with most of the girls shampooing and getting cleaned up for the formal scheduled that evening. Privacy was less than total in the shower rooms, and it was an all-hands-on-deck kind of undertaking to get more than a dozen campers showered and dressed in a short period of time.

I had seven campers left in the pool when I was called into the girl's bathroom. I turned the corner into the shower area and came face to face with Anna, a stark-naked and unhappy camper. Hands on her hips, she had planted her feet shoulder width apart and was pressing her lips tightly together. She was in her mid-twenties but looked much younger.

"Anna. What's up, my friend?" I faced her, my five-feet towering over her 4'9" frame.

"Stephanie won't take her bathing suit off." She stamped her foot as she said this, pointing at her counselor.

Stephanie held her hands up, clearly uncomfortable with the situation. "I tried telling her that staff can't be naked, but she doesn't believe me."

"I want her to be naked, and she won't do it!"

"You know what, Anna? Stephanie can't be naked. Campers can be naked, but staff absolutely cannot be naked. That's just the way it is."

"No! I want her to take off her bathing suit!" Anna wasn't budging, and Stephanie looked mortified. The campers and counselors were close in age during this session, so I could understand why Anna questioned the double standard.

I called out to Elizabeth, the assistant program director, who was in the corner shower, shampooing Ruby. "Elizabeth! Can counselors be naked?"

"Absolutely not. Campers yes, counselors no. That's just the way it is." Elizabeth had been listening and echoed my words, trying hard not to laugh.

Anna wasn't appeased. "Why? Why can't counselors be naked, Nurse Colleen?"

"Well, Anna, I know it doesn't seem fair, but my rule is that counselors have to keep their clothes on all the time. Naked is fine for campers, but for staff, it is just plain inappropriate. Sorry, but that's my rule."

Ruby chimed in from the shower. "Anna, staff has to be appropriate. Everyone knows that. They have all kinds of crazy rules. Aren't you getting cold standing out there with nothing on? Time's a wasting, girlfriend."

Elizabeth had her face turned to the wall, her shoulders shaking. A few more campers entered from the pool, heading towards the showers. Anna hadn't moved and appeared to be considering her options.

I tried redirection. "The shower next to Elizabeth and Ruby is free. Tonight is formal night, so you might want to wash your hair before we head back to camp. Maybe Stephanie will braid it for you. She's great with hair."

That got her attention. Anna looked at Stephanie, and she nodded. "I'd love to braid your hair, but we have to wash it first."

"Let's get moving— we don't have all day." Anna made a beeline for the shower, and Stephanie mouthed a "thank you" as she walked by. I made my way through the changing room, checking on campers as they dressed and making sure the counselors were okay.

I headed out to the pool, passing by the showers. Anna was talking to her friend Bethany, a fair-haired blonde who was covered in suds, still wearing her bathing suit. "You know, Bethany, you could take your suit off. Counselors have to keep their clothes on, but campers can be naked. That's the rules. I don't know about Nurse Colleen, though. Can nurses be naked?"

Without hesitation, Bethany offered one of my all-time favorite answers. "Nurses can do anything."

The pool was now empty, so I gathered my supplies to move out to the courtyard. I stopped outside the open door to the men's changing room, calling in to ask if everyone was okay. I heard a counselor call out to me. "You can come in if you want to, Nurse Colleen. We're decent."

A camper disagreed. "She can't come in here—she's a woman!"

"Nurse Colleen's not a woman! She's a nurse." I couldn't place the voice, but thought it might have been one of the counselors.

A wave of laughter rolled out of the men's room, colliding with the laughter coming from the girls. I stood between the doors, relishing the sound. Bobby, one of my morning coffee buddies, came out and offered to carry one of my bags. We walked out together, and when we got to the double doors that led outside, he opened a door for me, standing aside so I could pass.

"Nurses first."

I loved my job.

PRUNE PATROL

During staff orientation, I used catchy phrases and sheer repetition to imbed a few concepts into the minds of the counselors:

Your first question should always be, "Do you need to use the bathroom?"

If you're thirsty, your camper is thirsty.

If you are hot, your camper is hot.

Perspiring Pete says sweat is sweet, but if you're hot dry and red, look out kids you'll be dead!

If a camper runs away from the table during mealtime, follow them to make sure they aren't choking.

Always have an escape plan in the back of your mind. If you have to move a camper quickly, work with what you have. Know how you will do it.

I couldn't help but think of San Francisco when I talked about ways of moving people if you didn't have help. I showed them how you could wrap anyone in a sheet and pull them out of a tent or building.

I ended my training with a question for the counselors, "What do I want to know?"

"Everything! You want to know everything."

"Exactly. I need to know that everyone is eating, drinking, peeing, and pooping. If they aren't I can fix it, but I need to know."

I made rounds of all the tents each evening, checking in on every camper before they went to sleep and asking the counselors if there was anything I needed to know. I was especially vigilant with our older campers, making sure I added them to my prune patrol as soon as things "slowed down."

Every morning, I gave medications before breakfast. I had a little station built onto the porch of the lodge, right in front of the dining tents. At least 75% of my campers were on meds, and each one took them in their own unique way. Some were mixed in yogurt or applesauce, some were downed dry by the handful, some were taken one at a time, and some were chewed with gusto. Along with the supplies needed to give each camper's medications in the way that worked for them, I had a big bag of prunes, no prescription needed.

If anyone was feeling constipated, they joined my prune patrol. If they hadn't pooped for two days, they got put on prune patrol. Some of the counselors chose to put themselves on prune patrol. I put a few prunes in a paper soufflé cup and dispensed them along with morning meds.

There was one camper in particular, June, who was always focused on her bowels. As soon as she arrived at camp, she would tell me her stomach hurt, her abdomen was bloated, and she was constipated. It was a part of who she was, and I worked with her, checking her abdomen each evening, and making sure she was having bowel movements. She was a regular on the prune patrol.

On the very last morning of the session, June approached me looking very upset. She told me that she had had a "very big poop that pushed something out." She wanted me to check and make sure she was okay, and as we talked, she fidgeted, pulling at her shorts as if she had a wedgie.

We went into the bathroom by my office, and I took a peek. Sure enough, she had a few small hemorrhoids. I got her Preparation-H, put on my gloves, and as June phrased it, "put things back where they belonged."

As soon as the last camper left, I had to rush home for a meeting. One of my attorney-clients needed to discuss a report I had written the week before and was going to meet with his clients that evening. John was very supportive of my camp, attending fundraisers and asking lots of questions about camp life. He told me to come straight from camp and "not to worry if you look like you've been living in the woods all week."

I was still in camp nurse mode when I arrived and hadn't had time to switch gears back to legal nurse consultant. I took out a copy of my report, looked at my notes, and asked where he would like to start.

"I really need to understand what happened in the ER," he said. "What is it they should have noticed on the CAT scan?"

"Sure. To put it simply, she had a significant brain hemorrhoid that was clearly visible by CT scan."

His brow furrowed, and he looked puzzled. "A what?"

"A brain hemorrhoid," I repeated, still not catching my mistake.

"Are you sure about that, Colleen? A brain hemorrhoid?"

I started laughing. "Hem-o-rrhage, not hemorrhoid, hemorrhage! They missed an obvious bleed."

I lost it, laughing so hard tears ran down my face. John laughed right along with me, and he had one of those laughs that make you laugh harder. We were laughing so loudly that the receptionist came in to ask what was going on, telling us, "They can hear you all the way down the hall."

"Too bad," John said. "This is damn funny."

We finally made it through our discussion, and as I stood to leave he handed me a check, thanking me for a good job and a much needed laugh.

I was beyond punchy at that point, and since it was on my way home, I *literally* laughed all the way to the bank.

CHANGE OF COURSE

I did not get my happily-ever-after with Sean. After a year and a half together, it was clear we needed to be under separate roofs. I wasn't willing to settle for the purely platonic relationship that worked for him, and he wasn't looking for the fairy tale with me. I moved out of our home and once again considered my future.

In the summer of 2011, shortly after our split, Sean and I accomplished the monumental task of moving his parents (and my 2nd parents) from Wisconsin to Washington. Henry had metastatic lung cancer and had been given less than six months to live. Joan was in the moderate stages of Alzheimer's disease and needed lots of attention. The trip was harrowing, and Henry died in hospice just a week after we arrived. Sean and I took turns staying with Joan in her assisted living apartment while we waited for a bed to open in the memory care.

The experience with Sean, Joan, and Henry put me on a different path. It piqued my interest in hospice, and I became more involved in issues related to Alzheimer's/dementia. I wrote a book about our journey, which fulfilled a lifelong dream of being a writer. Seeing firsthand how important a support system was, I began blogging about caregiving and participating in online support forums.

Everything happens for a reason, and I believe I went to Washington so I could be reminded of what is truly important. I was given the opportunity to go back to camp, where I found new friends and much of the laughter I had been missing. Armed with fresh perspective, I left Washington in order to be closer to my family. I drove cross-country once again, intent on finding a way to combine all of my interests.

ROCKING

I arrived on the unit and introduced myself to Beth, the hospice nurse I had been told to ask for. She led me into a room and pointed to the rocking chair, saying, "That's where you'll be the most comfortable."

I settled into the chair, putting a pillow across my lap. Beth placed a ten-day-old baby in my arms, taking care not to disturb the dressing covering half of his scalp. Once he was comfortably settled on my lap, she asked, "Are you okay being left alone with him?"

"We'll be fine."

"Do you want me to start the CD before I leave?"

"No, thanks. I'm going to read to him." I opened my Kindle and hit the power button.

Beth smiled, "That's a new one. Call if you need me."

"I will." I looked at the list of titles I had downloaded and chose a classic Dr. Seuss. "Let's get started, shall we?"

And for two uninterrupted hours, I held a baby nearing end-of-life in my arms, rocking him gently and reading stories. It was something I had never had the opportunity to do as a nurse, but as a volunteer, I could just "be." This baby had been given a very short time on earth, and I felt privileged that I got to be a part of it, offering him a few hours of love, physical contact, and the sound of a human voice.

Over the course of ten days, I spent fourteen hours with this child, rocking him, reading to him, and telling him about the children that came before him. Joshua, who taught me to look down when I answered my door; Cindy, the reason I always started my questions with "Do you need to use the bathroom?"; and the campers who thought I was a decent alligator wrestler. I told him about Charlie, who thought his roommate was giving him the evil-eye, and Luke, the child I spent hundreds of hours with and never had the chance to rock.

Every time I finished my two-hour visit, the nurse thanked me for volunteering and for taking time out of my schedule. It was nice to be appreciated, but there was no doubt in my mind that I was the one on the receiving end. There was peace in that rocking chair.

TOMATO SANDWICHES

On a chilly Saturday morning, I walked into the assisted living facility to visit Dorothy, an eighty-six-year-old hospice patient with dementia. My time as a hospice volunteer was primarily spent with Alzheimer's and dementia patients. I would always find time to rock babies, but thankfully the need for that was infrequent. The need for visiting dementia patients would never slow down.

I had been visiting her for almost a year, but every time I visited, we met for the first time. As so often happens with dementia, her mood, awareness, and abilities varied day-to-day. I didn't know what I would find when I visited but had learned a few ways to better connect with her. As soon as I saw her, I knew she wasn't having a good day. She was picking at the seams of her quilt, moaning a little, and shaking her head back and forth as if to say "No."

I approached the end of her bed and introduced myself for the 45th time. "Hi, Dorothy. My name is Colleen, and I am a volunteer with hospice. May I sit with you for a few minutes?"

She didn't look up, remaining focused on the seams of her quilt, her movements almost suggesting she was sewing. I sat in the chair that was wedged between her bed and the window.

"It's really cold outside," I started. "You can see the frost on the ground."

"I wish they would get here," she said, briefly looking in my direction.

"Who are you waiting for?"

"My son. He's coming to take me home. I've been here a week since I broke my leg. They won't let me walk, but I am going home today." I knew that she had broken her leg when she was a teenager. Her son had told me that when I met him during one of my visits. He said she often thought a broken leg was the reason she was in the nursing home.

Dorothy had moved on to her bedside table, shifting items around and pulling handfuls of tissues from the box, crumpling them up and letting them fall onto her lap. "I can't find anything," she said in frustration. "Where are my keys?"

She looked unhappy, and I changed the subject to the only one that consistently brought her a measure of happiness. It was a topic we had discussed dozens of times before.

"Spring will be here before you know it, Dorothy. I can't wait to get back in my garden."

I didn't have her attention yet, so I continued. "There's nothing like pulling fresh vegetables from your garden, is there?"

"I grew the best tomatoes on the farm." It had worked, and she was engaged.

"What did you like to do with them?"

"Oh my, there is nothing like a tomato sandwich." A smile crossed her face. "Have you ever had one?"

"Do you mean a BLT?" Her hands stopped moving, no longer fidgeting with the tissues.

"No, ma'am, not at all. Just a plain tomato sandwich. There is nothing as good as a tomato sandwich made from your garden. Haven't you had one before?" She reached out and placed her hand on my forearm, apparently concerned that I had not enjoyed such a treat.

"I have had BLTs but not a plain tomato sandwich. How do you like to fix them?"

She closed her eyes and smiled. "You use plain white bread. Nothing fancy, just regular white bread from the store. You use mayonnaise, Duke's mayonnaise, not so much it's messy but don't be skimpy, either. You need enough so you know it's there. Add a little salt and pepper, thick slices of tomato, and you're done."

"That sounds wonderful," I said. "Nothing tastes as good as vegetables from your garden."

"I grow all kinds." Dorothy talked for about ten minutes, telling me about her vegetable garden back on the farm and offering a few tips on how to keep rabbits out of the garden. She abruptly stopped speaking and started picking at the seams of the quilt. "I think I want to close my eyes for a few minutes."

"Of course," I said, standing up. "I enjoyed talking with you, and if it's okay with you, I'll be back next Saturday."

"Stop by anytime, ma'am. I like having company."

I was halfway down the hall when I realized I had left my gloves on the window sill. I walked back into her room, and looked to see if she was sleeping. Her eyes were open, and as she turned towards me, I said, "Sorry to disturb you—I forgot my gloves."

She looked at me, confused. "Do I know you?"

GETTING BACK TO BUSINESS

I was on the phone with a new client and ended with the promise, "I'll give you the good, the bad, and the ugly, so you'll have the truth, the whole truth and nothing but the truth."

"So help me God," he said, finishing the phrase. "Hugh told me I would be happy with your work and that you send really good cookies at Christmas. I'll look forward to getting your report." He was hiring me to review a possible medical malpractice case, and my job was to give him the unvarnished truth about what had happened so he could make a decision about accepting or declining the case.

"Hugh does love a good cookie. I'll be in touch soon."

Hugh was an attorney I had been working with for eight years. I'd met his wife Ruth at a networking group in 2005, and when she heard my elevator speech, she handed me her husband's business card, saying "He'll have breakfast with you on Thursday." He did, I left with a case, and he has sent multiple clients my way. Over the course of eight years and more than one hundred cases, we had developed a friendship as well.

I hadn't expected friendships with clients when I started my business but have been fortunate to work with attorneys who are both excellent lawyers and genuinely nice people. By taking the time to get to know them, I was better able to tailor my work to their style and thought process. Out of the extra few minutes of chit-chat at the end of meetings, I got to know them, and they got to know me. Sometimes it led to a great working relationship, and other times, it led to a friendship born of common values and interests.

I wasn't friends with all my clients, of course, and had never met some of them. They were scattered across the country, and most often came to me by word of mouth recommendations from existing clients. There were two I had never even spoken with. They wanted to do everything by email, so we did. Messages in the middle of the night were not uncommon, and I did not envy their schedules.

I was writing a follow-up email to my new client when my phone rang. I smiled, seeing that it was a client in Washington State. We shared a deep devotion to the Chicago Bears and had commiserated over their last few seasons. While I lived in Washington, we had enjoyed frequent lunches and many, many laughs. A working relationship turned into a friendship I valued a great deal.

"Hi Brian," I said. "What's up?"

"Not much. The cases will be there next week sometime. I just wanted to see how you're doing and say hi. Did you watch Sunday's game?"

"Of course," I said. "And I'm sure this is the year we'll be doing the Super Bowl Shuffle. You doing okay?"

"Yep. Like I said, just wanted to say hello. Go Bears!"

"Go Bears." The important topic of the day covered, he hung up.

I looked around my home office. It was decorated with Bears paraphernalia, camp pictures, my rock collection from the beaches of Washington State, family photographs, artwork from my nephews, treasures collected during my years on the road, and an old unopened Coca-Cola bottle that had sat on my grandfather's desk for years.

"Go Bears," I said to the room. Life was good.

Epilogue:
Taking Root

When Maura and I discussed our dreams in Las Vegas, I told her that if I could build a successful business, it would give me time to pursue my passions. I wanted flexibility and freedom while making a comfortable living doing something I both liked and was good at. That is what legal nurse consulting has given me. It provides the freedom to work at camp in the summer, and the flexibility to change my day if something comes up.

As the years have passed, I've developed interests in divergent fields of nursing. Developmental disabilities, hospice, and Alzheimer's/dementia are all close to my heart, and since leaving Washington, I had expended a great deal of time and energy in trying to find a career path that would allow me to be active in all of these areas. In trying to figure out my next step, I reached out to my friends.

My grandmother once told me that if you went through life with a true friend you were lucky. If you had two, you were doubly blessed, and if you had three, you were more fortunate than most people on the planet. Louise, my roommate in Galveston, was one of those friends. She still is. Traveling placed a few more exceptional women in my path, and I became luckier than most people on the planet. Sam, my friend from the child psych unit in Boston, was now happily married and living in Chicago. Ann, my favorite traveling nurse, was now a nurse anesthetist and was still traveling. These were friendships unaffected by time and distance, the type that allow for honesty based on a true understanding of who I have always been.

A few months ago, I had lunch with Ann. Our lunches last hours as we reminisce about our adventures in San Francisco, laugh at what we did when we were young and foolish, and talk about our future dreams and aspirations. I told her I wanted to put down roots but still didn't think I had found where that was supposed to be. A lifelong traveler, she understood better than most the dilemma of having lived in too many places.

"The thing is, Ann, home is wherever my car is parked. There are good things and bad things in every place I have lived, and I can be happy anywhere. I take home with me."

"Well," she said, "I guess it comes down to a single question. When all is said and done, where do you want to park your car?"

"That simple, huh?"

"You said it—you can be happy anywhere. Your heart will tell you when you're home."

Follow your heart. It was the piece of advice I heard most often, coming from both family and friends. I took that advice and followed my heart back to Florida. When I drove across Tampa Bay, I once again felt the rush of excitement I had felt as a child on the way to my grandparent's house. Almost there, or, in my case now, almost home.

I do not know if Florida will be my final stop or if I will once again pack my car and start a new adventure. I certainly hope that my future will include many more summers at camp because it is the laughter, conversations and everyday moments spent with my campers that restore my faith in human nature.

Life continues to keep me guessing, and I have come to understand what a wonderful thing that is. It has been in unexpected places where I have found my greatest joys, and I know there is much more to come. There is no limit to what can be accomplished when focusing on things that truly matter, and I can make all of my interests a part of my life without making them a part of my job.

It took a little time for me to recognize that I don't have to be working as a nurse in order to *be* one. I can accept invitations to book clubs and use the time as an opportunity to start discussions on end-of-life and caregiving. As a hospice volunteer, I can visit dementia patients in nursing homes, and rock babies as they near end-of-life. In writing about my experiences with Alzheimer's disease, I try to let people know they aren't alone.

In all of these endeavors, it will be a lifetime of nursing that guides me. Years of traveling, families that allowed me to share their joys and sorrows, laughter among coworkers, campers that showed me true joy, and children I will never forget. When it comes right down to it, it doesn't matter where I am or what I am doing.

I am, always have been, and always will be a nurse.

ACKNOWLEDGEMENTS

I would like to offer special thanks to my family for their support and encouragement. I hope my brothers, sister, and six nephews will enjoy finding their names scattered throughout the story. It's my way of showing you are always on my mind, and if you happen to die or show up as a psychiatric patient, it is nothing personal!

To the patients and families who allowed me to be a part of their lives, I thank you. And to the campers and counselors who reminded me every single day how easy it is to find joy in simple moments, I will forever be grateful.

Liking the people you work with makes life much more pleasant, and to the clients who allowed me to know them well enough to become a friend, I am most appreciative.

I treasure the twisted sense of humor, unabashed laughter, unwavering support, and love I am given by my girlfriends. We have had a long and bumpy ride! From the bottom of my heart, I thank AW, MS, and LT for decades of friendship.

Writing doesn't have to be a solitary experience, and I was fortunate to join The Prose, a critique group that gave me honest, disparate, and helpful feedback that made for a clearer, more cohesive manuscript. Thank you, Caresse, for hearing my voice loud and clear.

Thanks to Kim and Karen for inviting me to join the *In Care of Dad* family. Having such a wonderful forum in which to share my stories was an unexpected and humbling gift. I truly respect what you are doing to help caregivers and their loved ones.

Finally, I would like to say thank you to the many, many nurses who taught me what to do, what not to do, and how to deal with the roller coaster that comes with a life in nursing. It is a ride well worth taking, and I wouldn't have missed it for the world.

CPSIA information can be obtained
at www.ICGtesting.com
Printed in the USA
BVOW08s1808031216
469705BV00002B/201/P